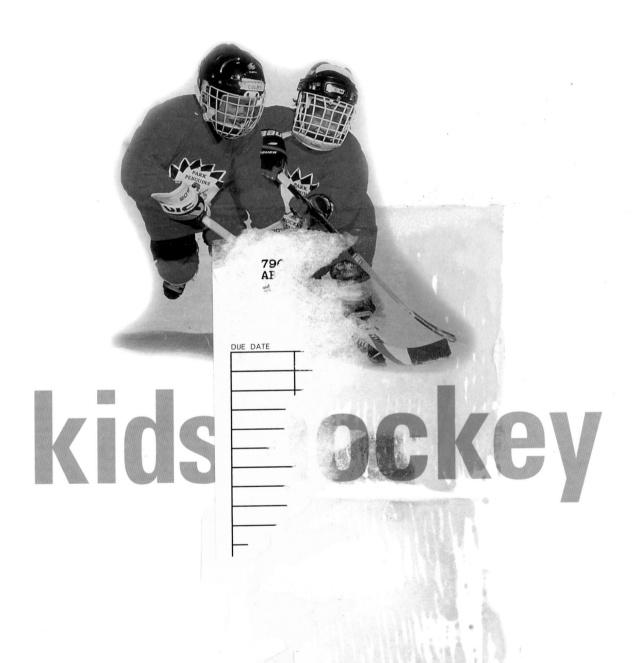

kids hockey

In memory of my brother, who loved the game.
Jason Joseph Abraham 1976–2000

For Mom, Dad, Kim and the boys

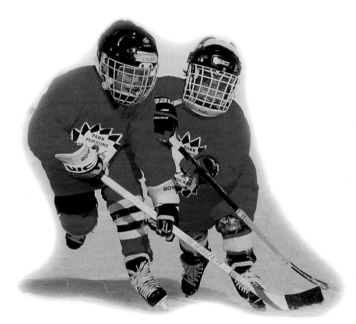

kids' hockey
THE PARENTS' GUIDE

GARY ABRAHAM, M.D.

with *Michael Smith*

FIREFLY BOOKS

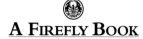

A FIREFLY BOOK

Published by Firefly Books Ltd. 2000

First Printing

U.S. Cataloging-in-Publication Data

Abraham, Gary.
     Kids' hockey : the parents' guide / by Gary Abraham.
−1st ed.
[176]p. : col. ill. ; cm.
Summary: Including hockey rules, skills, equipment,
safety, schools, rinks and organizations.
ISBN 1-55209-545-2
1. Hockey. 2. Hockey — Miscellanea. 3. National
Hockey League. I. Title.
796.962   21   2000   CIP

Canadian Cataloguing in Publication Data

Abraham, Gary
     Kids' hockey : the parents' guide

Includes bibliographical references.
ISBN 1-55209-545-2

1. Hockey for children. I. Smith, Michael, 1949- . II. Title.

GV848.6.C45A27 2000   796.962'083   C00-930876-8

Published in Canada in 2000 by
Firefly Books Ltd.
3680 Victoria Park Avenue
Willowdale, Ontario, Canada   M2H 3K1

Published in the United States in 2000 by
Firefly Books (U.S.) Inc.
P.O. Box 1338, Ellicott Station
Buffalo, New York, USA   14205

Design by Interrobang Graphic Design Inc.
Printed and bound in Canada by Friesens, Altona, Manitoba

The Publisher acknowledges the financial support of the Government of Canada through the Book Publishing Industry Development Program for its publishing activities.

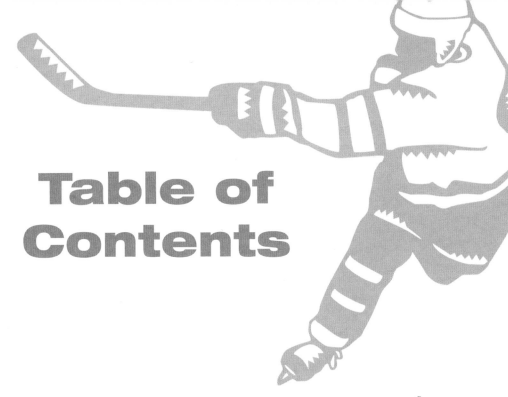

Table of Contents

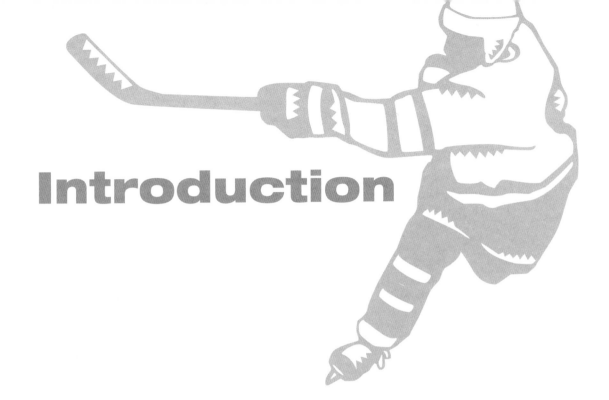

Introduction

HOCKEY IS GOOD FOR YOU

Hockey is fun, fast and great exercise. Played the right way, it's exciting and it's safe. As a doctor and a parent, I believe all children should play sports. Why? Well, it isn't just because of the coordination and physical well-being that sports help to develop. Equally important is the fact that team sports like hockey are a great way for your child to develop his or her social skills and to build self-esteem. Children with good self-esteem, who feel confident about themselves, are more likely to become successful adults. As parents we all want to see our children succeed in life. Our job is to get them into adulthood with as solid a base as we can provide. This includes the support and care they need at home, as well as experiences like team sports outside the home.

The great thing about hockey today is that it's a sport for both girls and boys. Young girls and boys often play on the same team nowadays. And if you happen to live in a community where there are enough kids, there may even be an all-girls' league.

I start by giving a brief history of the game. I also give a complete review of the rules of the game, so you'll understand what is happening on the ice and can figure out those signals that the referee keeps making. If you don't know anything about the game, then this book will fill you in. But even experienced hockey parents should find a lot of useful information here. Do you know how to make sure skates fit? How to tape a stick? How to size a goalie stick properly? Why some penalties are "good" and others aren't? If not, then read on—you'll find all that information here and much, much more.

If you have some reservations about your child playing ice hockey, don't feel alone. It's our job as parents to worry. Read this book and you'll be taking great strides toward becoming a very confident hockey parent. I have been involved in hockey for 30 years. I know that played the right way hockey is safe, and I have yet to meet a child who doesn't enjoy the game. Not only that, hockey is a great and exciting sport for the parents to watch.

If you're concerned about safety, I will teach you all about the equipment and how to outfit your child correctly—from the right helmet to properly fitted skates. If you're a parent who has already played the game, I know you will find some useful tips here, particularly in the equipment chapters. Believe me, the game and the equipment are very different from when we played as kids. Is your child a goalie, or thinking about playing goal? I've devoted a whole chapter to the equipment and the special role this player has on the team.

But this book is not only about equipment and safety. Basic hockey skills and how to teach them form a substantial part of my approach to hockey. I'm a big believer in basic skills over complex strategy—particularly when the kids are just starting out. Even if you've never worn a pair of skates, I'll show you ways to help your child improve. I've included lots of exercises and basic skills that can be practiced on and off the ice. If you're thinking about sending your child to a hockey school but aren't sure how to go about it, I discuss this in Chapter 9. I even give you my secret formula for how to build a backyard rink. If you are interested in coaching or becoming a referee, I discuss these topics in the appendixes. I've also included lists of resources on children's hockey organizations as well as lots of other great stuff—from educational websites to videos on puck-handling.

Let's talk more specifically about the genuine concerns and fears that parents might have about their child playing hockey. I offer my thoughts on this as a medical doctor, a coach, and a parent of three young players.

Many new hockey parents are concerned about safety and body-checking. Let me assure you that body-checking doesn't start until the age of 12 at the earliest, and in most regular or house leagues it is not allowed at all. However, hockey does involve body contact, and I provide some tips you can pass on to your child on how to play smart (see the section on Body Contact and Checking in Chapter 3). The bottom line is hockey in the early years is very safe. The worst injury you're likely to see, if the child is properly equipped, is a bruise. (I give an overview of injuries and safety in Chapter 7, Hockey Health and Safety.)

If you are worried that hockey is too violent a game for your child, I can also assure you that what you see on TV is nothing like a children's ice hockey game. When they are starting out, most kids are worried about keeping themselves on two feet, not about retaliating for a hard body-check. Nonetheless, kids' hockey is strictly regulated. Fighting and other forms of aggressive activity are absolutely forbidden. In fact, many children's leagues have a zero-tolerance rule for violence. At minimum, overly aggressive players are removed from the game. I discuss this further in Chapter 2 and in Appendix 2.

Is ice hockey expensive? Well, there is no doubt you can spend a lot of money on equipment. However, this book will show you how to make smart choices when it comes to your child's equipment. With some exceptions, used equipment is often perfectly satisfactory, and I provide you with some tips on making sure it will do the job for your child. The idea here is to make the game affordable to you as a parent. Sure, it costs money to sign up your child. But remember that this money pays for ice time, uniforms and referees.

Time. There is no question that hockey requires a certain amount of time and commitment on your part. But that is true of any youth sport. Yes, you'll have to get up early some mornings. If there's a tournament, you might spend part of the day in a rink. But believe me, it's cheaper than a trip to the mall. Supporting your child at the rink shows that you're involved in his or her interests and activities. It's a simple way to help build self-esteem. And not only do the kids develop new relationships with other players and the coaches, but—and I've seen this time and again—hockey parents form great friendships in the stands as they attend the games and practices over the season.

Many of you reading this book are single parents. Single parents are often extremely busy and under a great deal of pressure at home. It can be hard to make it to all the games and practices. Does this mean you should keep your child out of hockey? No. Almost any child will understand that you can't make it to *all* the games and practices. As for transportation, informal car-pooling is a big part of kids' hockey. I talk about these issues in Chapter 8, Good Hockey Parenting.

In the last few years there have been some high-profile incidents of sexual abuse in hockey. This is a legitimate concern, but from my experience as a coach with very young players it isn't likely to happen, mainly because for the first two or three years of hockey the dressing rooms are so full of parents and players that nothing *could* happen. However, I do give attention to this important issue in Chapter 8.

These are all important issues. It would be foolish to pretend they aren't genuine concerns. But a kid's early years in hockey should be a great experience, full of fun, learning, growth and excitement. This book was written to give parents everything they need to make that happen.

I'm sure you are wondering what makes me such an expert on children's ice hockey. Well, I have been involved in the game for many years as a medical doctor, player, coach and referee, and as an instructor at my own hockey school. Not only that, I'm the father of three budding players—Brayden, Spencer and Bryce.

I've been practicing family and sports medicine since 1991 and have lots of experience looking after children. I am also a partner with the Sports Medicine Specialists, a clinic dedicated to sport injuries and the high-performance training of athletes. Our organization looks after the Toronto Maple Leafs of the NHL, and the Brampton Battalion and St. Michael's Majors who play in the Ontario Hockey League, the premier Junior league in the world. As the team physician for the Brampton Battalion, I spend many hours in the rink looking after the hockey stars of tomorrow.

As a hockey player I played my minor hockey in Chinguacousy, in what is now called the Brampton Youth Hockey Association, one of the largest hockey associations in the world. My career as a player ended at the University of Waterloo, where I was a member of the varsity hockey team, the Waterloo Warriors. While I played hockey, I also refereed in the Ontario Minor Hockey Association. Since I've long been interested in children's hockey, I obtained my Level 3 referee certification in 1980 and have been involved in refereeing minor hockey at all levels and ages.

As the owner and director of the Albion Hills Hockey School (in Caledon, Ontario), I've been teaching children ages 6 to 12 every summer since 1982. I try to help kids play better hockey and let them have fun while they do it. But so often I've seen kids in equipment that wasn't safe or didn't fit properly. In fact, repeatedly seeing the poor choices parents have made in purchasing equipment was one of the main reasons for writing this book. Kids feel more comfortable, play better and are safer when they're wearing good, well-fitted equipment.

When my children were old enough to play in a league, I started my coaching career. In the last five years I have coached kids at all levels from ages 4 to 9. To become a certified coach I took courses endorsed by the Canadian Hockey Association.

As a parent, I have three boys involved in hockey. The two oldest, Brayden and Spencer, play representative (or all-star) hockey. Bryce is too young for a league, but comes out to my team's practices or skates for hours on our backyard rink. So with three boys playing, I have had lots of experience in selecting equipment and know what works and what doesn't. As a doctor, I have no reservations about my children playing the game because I know it's safe.

Kim, my wife of over 10 years, is a stay-at-home mom. She helps out tremendously with the hockey and has really grown to love the game. Kim has also made some good friends along the way. Both of us have great times going to the tournaments and the social functions that happen around hockey, such as dances and team parties. Hockey does get you out of the house. As well as hockey, we all enjoy skiing in the winter. And in summer the kids are into baseball, swimming and lacrosse. We feel that sports are an important way of promoting health, fitness and togetherness.

I'd like to thank Michael Smith, an award-winning Toronto journalist, who helped to sift through my many drafts and bring order to my sentences. Michael is an experienced hockey parent himself and his two sons, David and Robin, still enjoy the game. As a final note, I'd also like to thank my editor, Kent Enns, who took a real interest in trying to give shape and style to my first book.

Hockey has been a lifelong source of joy for me, and with my wife I have tried to pass that on to our children. We hope this book will make it easier for you to do the same.

CHAPTER 1

The Origins of Hockey and How It's Organized Today

A BIT OF HISTORY

You have to walk before you can run, the old saying goes, and similarly you have to skate before you can play hockey. The first skates were made of animal bones (the word "skate" means shank or leg bone), but it wasn't until iron skate blades were invented in the 1500s that skating became popular as a winter activity. Not long after, some European field games—such as hurley, played with a curved stick and ball—were being played on the smooth surfaces of frozen canals and lakes. By the 17th century just about every European country with a climate cold enough to freeze water played ice games that we might think of as precursors to modern hockey.

As the game of hockey evolved in the 19th century, it was played on frozen ponds and lakes. The rules were probably very informal—much different from modern hockey—and, indeed, might vary from town to town. It wasn't until the late 1800s that the first formal leagues, with established rules of play, came into being.

The first direct ancestor of our modern game took place in Canada near the end of the 19th century, although there's still a debate about where exactly the first games were played: Halifax, Montreal and Kingston, Ontario, have all been credited. It's now generally accepted that the first organized hockey game was played in 1875 at McGill University in Montreal. It was organized by James Creighton, a Halifax engineer whom many call the father of organized ice hockey. He brought the idea for the game and the rules with him from the Maritime provinces, where the modern game probably had its roots. Hockey then spread through eastern Canada, slowly made inroads into the United States (likely through Boston, with its longstanding connection to the Maritimes) and eventually reached western Canada.

That first game didn't much resemble a modern National Hockey League game. There were nine players on each team, and they all played the entire game with no protective equipment. The goals were marked by four-foot poles, spaced six feet apart, with a goal umpire who stood nearby and rang a bell when the puck crossed the line. The goalkeeper wasn't allowed to sit or sprawl across the ice, but on the other hand the puck could not be raised and no forward passing was allowed. For the skaters, the name of the game was stick-handling; they had to outmaneuver their opponents to get down the ice because they couldn't pass ahead. The single referee couldn't call penalties, but could throw a player out if he played too roughly.

The game was brought inside sometime in the 1870s—well after the first covered ice surfaces were created for recreational skating. By the early 1900s, covered ice surfaces or arenas were popping up all over North America, and shortly afterward artificial ice was developed in the United States. This development meant hockey could, in principle, be played throughout the year. But the technology was expensive and most games continued to be played on natural ice well into the 1940s and 1950s. Indeed, for many players and fans, the backyard rink or the neighborhood pond remains a powerful symbol of their childhood.

The National Hockey League added blue lines in 1918 and allowed forward passing within each defensive zone. In 1943 the center (or red) line was introduced and passing from one zone to the next was allowed (except for the off-side pass; see Chapter 2 for rules). With the center red line, the game entered what is referred to as its modern age. But the object of the game has always been the same: to get the puck in the other team's net. In the early years of hockey some pucks were made of wood or whatever else was handy. Vulcanized rubber was invented in 1839, but it took until the 1880s for it to be used in pucks. Even then pucks were just layers of rubber laminated together. Naturally they tended to fall apart. Today's solid rubber puck is the same size as 100 years ago—a 3-inch disk, 1 inch high—and weighs 5½ to 6 ounces. The Canadian Hockey Association, by the way, recently announced that it would like to see Novices (9 years old or younger), play with 4-ounce pucks.

When hockey was first starting on frozen lakes and ponds, anyone could play and anyone did. As men's hockey was becoming organized, so was women's. But there were few women's teams, so it was hard for young girls to play. Still, before World War II, women's hockey flourished; there was even a Canadian championship. But after the war, interest in the women's game diminished, making it difficult for young girls to find a team to play on.

Today, the situation is radically different. Girls' and women's hockey are growing fast. A lot of the increased growth in girls' hockey is due to the Women's World Championship, first held in 1990. But the greatest boost was the 1998 Winter Olympic Games in Nagano, Japan, where women's hockey finally became an Olympic medal sport. It was nice to see a North American team (the United States) win the gold medal.

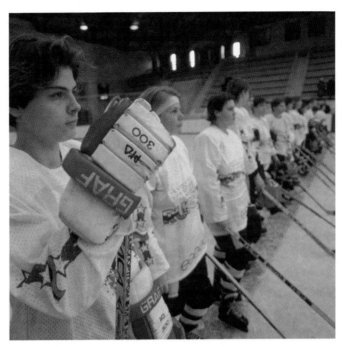

The Olympics and the world championships have given women's hockey a high profile.

Today, well over a million kids play hockey in North America. The game has become a large part of our culture. Players in the NHL are heroes to many of our children (and us). Ironically, the great success of many professional players and the widespread popularity of the NHL are among the greatest dangers to kids' hockey. The amount of money in the game at its highest levels is staggering. This sometimes blinds people to the fact that hockey really is just a game. And if you're a parent, always remember that it's a game for your child. The less you are caught up with winning and competitiveness, the more you and your child will enjoy this great game.

GETTING STARTED WITH YOUR LOCAL ASSOCIATION

So your child wants to play hockey—the first year in a new sport. There are lots of questions, but one of the most basic is this: How do you find a team?

The easiest way is to go to your nearest arena and ask about kids' hockey. Either the rink will have a program or the arena manager will know where the office of the nearest hockey association is. (Often such offices are right in the rink.) You can also ask neighbors, friends and family. Or look in the phone book. Very often, local hockey associations send around a flyer to remind parents of their hockey programs. Hockey is a popular sport, and it should be fairly easy to find information.

But because hockey is popular, space is often limited. So, timing is important—you can't just walk in the door as soon as the leaves fall and expect to have your son or daughter on the ice that winter. You might be lucky, but don't count on it. Plan ahead and make sure your child is registered in time for this first year of hockey. Some associations start registering as early as April or May for the following winter season.

The cost of registration varies widely from association to association, but it will probably be a couple of hundred dollars. The cost covers ice time, payment for referees, a team sweater and team socks. If your child is good enough to make a rep (or all-star) team—about which more later—there will be additional costs.

Your local hockey association will follow the guidelines set by a national organization (either USA Hockey or the Canadian Hockey Association). Each local association oversees and organizes registration, age groups, numbers of teams, ice time, coach selection, officials (referees and timekeepers) and tournaments. The association will have a convenor for each age group. This person supervises coaches and officials (by watching games), and acts as a liaison between the local executive board and the teams (including coaches, players and parents). If you have problems or concerns about your child's team, coaching or anything else, you can talk to the convenor, who will be able to give you more information and if necessary represent your concerns to the association executive.

GIRLS IN HOCKEY

Fifteen years ago, when I started running a hockey school, I would have said you were crazy if you had suggested that girls and boys could play hockey together. But you have to remember, even 15 years ago it was rare for men and women or girls and boys to play *any* sport together. At the hockey school, it was a nonissue—no one ever asked, and I never gave it a second thought.

Like all of us, I've changed a bit since then. I now think it's great for girls and boys to play hockey together—at least in the early years—and I don't see any real problems. After all, the kids are playing hockey to have fun, socialize and build self-esteem. And sometimes in a family we do too many separate activities, going our separate ways. It's nice to have an activity where the whole family—boys, girls and parents—can participate.

I don't have any first-hand experience as a parent with girls and hockey, because all my children are boys. But both as a coach and at my hockey school, I've seen many girls play the game. One year, my middle son's team—which I coached—had four girls. What was interesting to me was that I never noticed the difference: They were all just kids having fun.

To my mind, the kids themselves don't have a problem. Sure, most young boys will frown and make a face if they're asked about girls playing hockey, but once they get on the ice, the differences fade and they all just play the game. Parents, on the other hand, sometimes do have concerns. Will the boys play too rough? Will their girl fit in? And they sometimes prefer a girls' league, if they can find one.

With one exception, the rules are the same for the girls' and boys' game. The exception is that in girls' hockey, no matter what age group, intentional body-checking is not allowed. With older players you'll see a lot of contact, especially in the Olympics or national championships, because it is still permitted to ride an opponent off the puck. But intentional body-checks are penalized. On the other hand, girls who play on a boys' team—once they're at a level where body-checking is allowed—play by those rules. But none of this should matter if you are the parent of a girl who is just starting hockey. In all likelihood body-checking will not be allowed—for boys or girls. By the way, there are only a couple of differences between hockey equipment for young girls and boys. I talk about that in Chapter 4.

For my money, the time for a specialized girls' league is later, once the boys start to muscle up and become more aggressive. For the young kids, there's not much difference in size and strength— or if there is, it's not because of their gender. In fact, at some points in their development, the girls, by and large, are going to be bigger and stronger than the boys.

And let's face it, ice time is at a premium in North America and should be treated as a scarce resource. The best arrangement, I think, is one that allows the most kids to play.

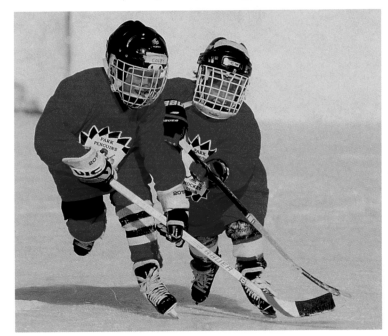

Mite Girls and Boys Playing Together
Below the age of 10 years, there are few differences in size and strength between boys and girls.

Finding a Team for Your Girl

As you'll have gathered, my feeling is that your best bet is to let your daughter play on whatever team is available, especially in her first few years as a hockey player. But if you do find an all-girls' league, you may discover that the teams are organized by skill level. In other words, there are no age categories, which may mean your 7-year-old beginner is playing against much older girls who are also beginners. This is not universal, but it's one way of making the best of a smaller pool of players.

Your daughter may be a gifted athlete and want to play at a higher level. Again, it will be easier for her to find a select or all-star program within the mixed children's hockey program. If you live in a small town or rural area, you may have to drive to the city to find a girls' league with an all-star program. Given that all-star hockey usually means at least two games and a practice every week, you could find yourself on the road a lot.

Playing on a Mixed Team

Kids don't usually have a problem with mixed teams. But there is one complication: the locker room. Traditionally, that's where the players change, with lots of shouting and joking. The locker room is where a lot of the camaraderie of the team is built. My co-author Mike has a son Robin who is always the first into the dressing room and the last out—and he's talking the whole time. The dressing room is a key part of the whole hockey experience, in my view.

But the tradition runs into problems when the teams are mixed. Hockey rinks are not designed to have separate dressing rooms for boys and girls. And such a separation would cut out a central part of the whole experience—trading jokes, teasing teammates and just letting off steam.

Some kids—boys and girls—are bashful about changing in front of others, especially others of the opposite gender. Many parents solve the problem by having their child come to the rink already in long underwear or with the inside layers of equipment already on. In this way modesty is preserved and so is the team experience. Also, you may find your daughter is the only girl on a mixed team. It is important that she doesn't show up five minutes before the game to put on her skates; she'll miss out on a lot of the fun. Being the only girl on the team usually isn't a problem but I would worry a bit if I heard some of the boys teasing others by comparing them unfavorably to her. Something like: "You're awful! Even Emily is better than you." This sort of thing—which is rare, I'm happy to say—needs to be nipped in the bud, by the coach and parents. All the players are teammates; they need to learn that teammates don't disparage each other.

One last thing. Most coaches are men. Why? Because coaches are volunteers and the people who volunteer are usually those with some hockey knowledge. Mostly those people are dads with kids in the program.

But there's no reason why Mom can't volunteer as well. Every team needs assistant coaches, whose main job is really to open the doors to the players' bench and to keep order on the bench. It's nothing too taxing and you don't really need to know much about the game. (If you do volunteer and come to like it, you can always take a coaching course and become a head coach.)

Having a woman—or even an older girl—as part of the coaching staff is a great idea for mixed teams. The boys have all sorts of role models. Why not a few for the girls?

AGE GROUPS

Kids' hockey is divided into classes, based on age. In the United States, the key is the age of the child on June 30; in Canada it's December 31. When you sign your child up, the local association will need to see his or her birth certificate (or other such proof of identity). In general, kids start to play at about age 5 or 6, and they're placed on Initiation or Beginner teams. The names of the age classifications vary a bit from place to place and association to association, but the following are pretty standard:

Initiation or Beginner	5 and under
Pre-Tyke or Mini-Mite	6 and under
Tyke	7 and under
Novice or Mite	9 and under
Atom or Squirt	11 and under
Peewee	13 and under
Bantam	15 and under
Midget	17 and under

The first three levels are single-year categories, but the higher levels cover more than one year. Usually, hockey associations will divide the upper levels. The Atom level, say, will be split into Minor Atom (the 10-year-olds) and Major Atom (the 11-year-olds). But if there aren't very many kids signed up for a level, the two age groups in it may be mixed.

In the first few years, girls will usually play with boys. All-girls' teams start to appear about the Minor Peewee level—the 12-year-olds—although there are more and more leagues for girls starting at the Tyke level.

At the Beginner level, kids are first introduced to hockey. The emphasis at this age is on fun and safety, but full equipment is required. Usually, they can already skate; if your child can't, you'd probably do best to postpone hockey for a year and sign him or her up for a learn-to-skate program.

At the Pre-Tyke level, some associations start mini games, but with few formal rules. Skating is the major skill that's emphasized. By this time, some kids are getting quite good at handling the puck.

Unfortunately, in my view, hockey starts to get too serious too soon. At the Tyke level, games become more formal, with referees and full rules. Many children have a tough time adjusting. This is also the age group when the first rep teams (more later) are formed.

At the Novice level, the children are really improving their skills, although there is often a huge discrepancy between players. About this time, the games become more competitive.

Some associations allow body-checking at the Atom level, although usually only on rep teams. Skill levels are still very uneven. By now, some of the kids have played together for several years and are forming strong friendships.

At the Peewee level, we suddenly see differences in the physical size of the kids, as puberty hits some and not others. The differences can be as much as 50 pounds and 10 inches. Body-checking is typically allowed on the rep teams, and may be allowed in house leagues. For some, the game is becoming very competitive—often this comes from parents or coaches, with the sad result that more kids start quitting at this age.

Bantam-level players are at a nice age—they can dress themselves and sometimes even get themselves to the rink. They're also bigger, so the physical aspect of the game—with its attendant risks—becomes more important.

Midget players love the game. They have to—anyone who doesn't love hockey has fallen by the wayside before reaching this level. At this age, they understand teamwork and some are good enough to play Junior hockey and maybe even dream of a major-league career.

Junior hockey is for players between 16 and 20 and is divided into levels according to the caliber of play.

TEAM CATEGORIES: HOUSE LEAGUE, SELECT AND REP

Now, I've been making a distinction between ordinary hockey (or house league) teams and what are called rep or all-star teams. These two main categories of teams at any age are based on skill level. The house league takes all the kids who sign up, divides them into teams and has them play against each other, usually at a set time and almost always at the same arena. But there may also be a local rep team—so called because it "represents" the local community. Such teams typically compete against rep teams from other communities, which means there is often much more travel involved. They also tend to play in more tournaments.

The players must try out to make a rep team. Understandably, they tend to have better skills than most of the kids in house league. If the child makes the rep team, those skills tend to improve more quickly, because the rep players get better coaching, more ice time and more practice time. You should also be aware that while the stated goals of amateur hockey at this level are still fun and self-esteem, the emphasis on competition is usually higher with rep teams.

You may hear people talk about "single-A" or "double-A" rep teams. This refers to the classification—by skill level—of the teams. A big city, such as Chicago or Toronto, will have teams at all levels; a smaller city, with a smaller talent pool, will have teams at fewer levels. By having more divisions according to skill level within each age group, different hockey associations in different communities can arrange to have more evenly matched teams playing against each other. This makes a big difference at tournaments, when a team of double-A caliber would otherwise clean up against 10 other rep teams at the single-A level.

As should be clear by now, the rep teams play against other rep teams, and their playing schedule can be hectic. It's not uncommon for a rep team to play two games a week, in widely separated arenas, and also to practice twice a week. They'll also play weekend tournaments, with as many as five or six games in three days.

But that's not the whole story. Between the rep teams and house league there's yet another level, called select. These intermediate-level teams are formed from the best of the remaining house league players. The select team will play against other select teams from other leagues, but the kids will also keep playing on their house league teams. They may also play in a few weekend tournaments.

Like the rep teams, select teams practice more, play more games and develop their hockey skills faster than in house league. While the skill level is lower than in rep teams, the emphasis on competition will probably be greater than in house league.

For parents, rep or select means more time spent in chilly arenas, sipping bad coffee. It's also going to cost more, although it's impossible to say how much since the costs vary widely even within associations. Just to give you an idea, though, consider that the higher fees go toward getting more than twice as much ice time. As well, the tournaments cost money—some charge as much as $1,000 a team, which has to be paid for by the parents. Many rep teams find sponsors or have raffles at the beginning of the season to help offset tournament and ice-time expenses.

For some kids, rep or select may turn out to be too much hockey, which can interfere with things like homework and piano practice.

But I don't want to be pessimistic. If your child is good enough to make a rep or select team, give it a shot. It can turn out to be a great experience, both for you and your young player. I have two boys playing rep hockey and the third is in the wings. As a consequence, my wife and I have made many new friends. And the sheer fun the kids have at a tournament is wonderful to behold. Just be aware that rep or select hockey is a big commitment.

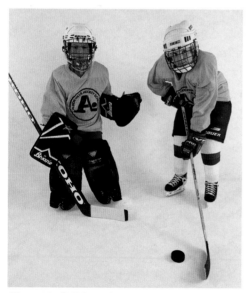

Players in Full Gear
My boys, Brayden and Spencer, fully dressed to play. The equipment allows for freedom of movement while protecting the kids from injury. Spencer's the goalie.

COMPOSITION OF THE TEAM

In kids' hockey, most teams have 16 or 17 players, usually nine forwards, six defense and one or two goalies. Some teams may have fewer players, depending on how many children are registered for hockey in that area.

Only six players per team are allowed on the ice at any one time. Usually, one of these players is the goaltender. But it can happen that during the game the coach will pull the goalie and put on an extra skater—either to try to tie the score late in the game or to take advantage of a delayed penalty. (I'll discuss this later).

The three basic positions in ice hockey are goaltending, defense and forward.

The goaltender's job is to keep the puck out of the net. Goaltenders wear special equipment—oversized shin pads, extensive shoulder and arm padding and specialized gloves—and they also use a different stick than the rest of the players. This equipment is much more expensive than the gear for the other players. For that reason, most kids' leagues will have a supply of goal equipment that is given out before each game.

Goaltending is by far the hardest position to play in hockey. When children are first learning to play, coaches will often allow each player to try the position. Some kids just take naturally to the position, while others struggle. But it's important for all kids to play goal at least once—it gives them a better idea of how difficult it is. You'll sometimes hear kids in the dressing room complaining about their goalie; this is unfair, and as a parent you should squelch such talk. Everybody makes mistakes, but the goalie's mistakes go up in lights on the scoreboard.

Goaltending responsibilities are usually spread around in the first two or three years of hockey. It's best that a child, even if he or she wants to play goal, learns skating and puck-handling before specializing. Once committed to the net, the goalie will focus on developing skills only goalies need

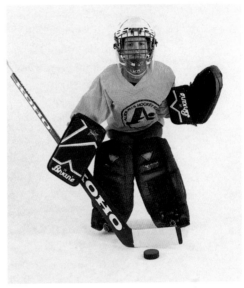

Goaltender in Full Gear
The goalie wears special equipment for protection.

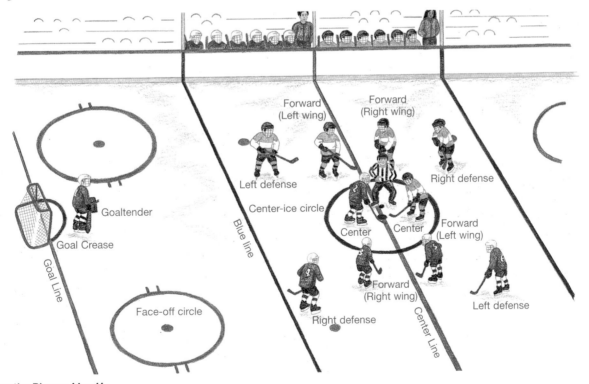

How the Players Line Up
Positions in hockey are fluid. The positions are named for the way the players line up on face-offs.

to know. Sometimes a coach will regularly put one of the weaker skaters in goal—which isn't fair. That child's skating will improve more out of the net than in. The position should be rotated.

There are three forwards—the left-winger, the center and the right-winger. The positions are named for the way they line up on a face-off; there's no rule that says the right-winger, for example, can't skate over to the left wing if the play goes that way.

The main job for the forwards is scoring. They're usually strong skaters who can cover a lot of ice quickly. And they have to—they sometimes need to get from behind the other team's goal line back into their own end in time to help out the defense and then help take the puck back up the ice on the attack.

There are two defense players, one on the left side and one on the right. The defense pair—especially if they're good—are the quarterbacks of the play. They usually have the puck when the team is breaking out of its own zone on the attack. A good defense player is a good skater, both forward and backward, has a cool head and can make a good pass to a streaking forward.

The main jobs of the defense are to prevent goals by breaking up the opposition's attack and to gain possession of the puck in the defensive zone and move it up to the forwards.

In the first few years of hockey, your child's team will probably use a buzzer system to change players. The buzzer will go off (usually while your child has a breakaway!), and all five skaters will change. Each shift will last (depending on how your league does things) for two or three minutes. This system is used for two reasons: to make sure that all the kids get the same amount of ice time, and because in the first few years they're not coordinated enough to change on the fly.

Changing on the fly—without waiting for a whistle—usually starts at the Atom (11-year-old) level, although your league may do things differently. In all-star or rep hockey, no matter what age, players will change on the fly, and as the kids get older all leagues eventually use the system. This doesn't mean coaches can't wait for a stoppage in play and change then. As often as not, players change after the referee blows his whistle. Changing on the fly has its dangers, including getting a penalty for having too many players on the ice. The substitute player can go on only after the player coming off the ice is within 10 feet of the bench.

Hockey is the only sport where players are allowed to substitute without a stoppage in play. It's also an extremely fast game, in which players tire quickly. By the time your child is 12 or 13, shifts will have dropped from two minutes to one minute or even less. In the NHL, shifts are often shorter than 30 seconds.

For these first few years, however, it's convenient to let the clock decide when it's time to come off the ice. Many kids have trouble with short shifts; they complain to the coach or to their parents that they just get going when they have to come off. There will come a time (if your child sticks with hockey for a few seasons) when you'll need to point out that a player is of little use to the team when playing without the "jump." Floating around the ice instead of letting someone with fresh legs play is unfair to the rest of the team.

Until then, you'll have enough to worry about: getting your child signed up for the season, let alone getting him or her to practices and games. As for following all the rules and referee signals, I discuss them next.

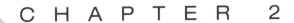

CHAPTER 2

Playing the Game
The Rules

THE GAME TODAY

Because a well-played game of hockey is so fast, many people—especially those who haven't grown up with the sport—find it hard to follow. But the basic idea is simple: Put the puck in the other team's net, while stopping them from putting it in yours. Naturally, there's more to it than that, but if you bear that objective in mind, you'll soon understand many of the other rules. If you already understand the game, by the way, feel free to skip ahead to the chapters on skills or equipment.

First things first. A hockey rink is divided into sections by lines on the ice. There's a center red line, which divides the ice into two parts. On each side of the center red line is a blue line. The blue lines divide the ice roughly into thirds. And near either end (about 11 feet from the end boards) is a thin red line called the goal line. On the goal line is—you guessed it!—the goal net, which is six feet wide and four feet high.

A goal is awarded when the puck *completely* crosses the goal line and enters the net. As you'd expect, the team with the most goals at the end of the game wins. In most leagues, teams get two points for a win, one for a tie and none for a loss. If a winner must be declared—in playoffs, for instance—teams will play sudden-death overtime periods in which the first team to score a goal wins. (National Hockey League teams play a five-minute sudden-death overtime period if a game is tied at the end of regulation time. But if no one scores during the five minutes, the game ends in a tie. The NHL recently added a new wrinkle to the point system. Both teams get a point if regulation time ends in a tie, but if a team wins in overtime, it gets another point. This is intended to encourage the teams to play all-out during the overtime.)

A professional or Junior game is divided into three 20-minute periods, with a short (usually 15-minute) break between each period. The clock stops when play stops, which is why major league hockey games can sometimes take up to three hours.

In kids' hockey, the rules vary. Some leagues let the clock run; they've budgeted an hour's ice time for the game and stopping the clock would run them over budget. Others use stop-time only for part of the game—the last two minutes, for example—or only when the game is close. Also kids' games are usually shorter—perhaps three 10-minute periods or even one 30-minute period. As the players get older, the length of games increases.

A few other details. The players (when they're not on the ice) sit on either the visitors' bench or the home team's bench. There'll usually be a sign to tell you which is which. (And usually the home team will wear white jerseys and the visitors will wear colors.) There's also a penalty box and a booth for the timekeeper, who starts and stops the clock and writes down who got penalties and who scored and when. There may also be goal judges at either end of the ice, behind the net (but off the ice), whose job it is to turn on a red light when the puck enters the net.

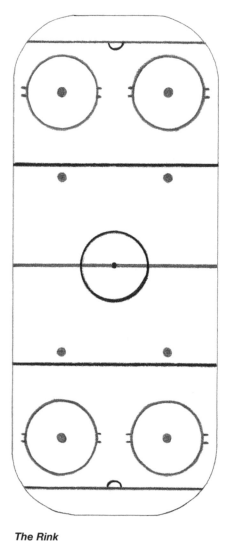

The Rink

Rink markings are standard, from your local ice surface to the National Hockey League.

Recall I said there are five lines on the ice (one red center, two blue and two goal). A quick glance will show you there is actually a lot more than that. For instance, in front of each goal is an area of blue (or sometimes white) ice enclosed in a red line. This is the goal crease, a "safe" zone, in which the goaltender is supposed to be immune from deliberate contact by other players. (You'll recognize the goaltender immediately by the big awkward-looking pads, the large flat stick and the oversized gloves.)

About 60 feet from the goal lines are the blue lines, which divide the ice into three zones—the defensive, offensive and neutral zone. If you hang around hockey rinks, you'll hear coaches, players and fans talk about "getting the puck out of the zone." They mean getting the puck out of their team's defensive zone, which is the area between their goal and the nearest blue line. Naturally, one team's defensive zone is the other team's offensive zone. Another thing you'll hear is coaches and fans yelling at players to "clear the zone." That means to get out of the offensive zone and avoid an off-side (about which more later).

In each zone are a number of red dots. These are where the puck will be put back in play—"faced off"—after a stoppage. Most face-offs will take place at the red dots enclosed in red circles (there are four of them; two at either end of the rink), but face-offs to start the game and each period and after each goal take place at the blue dot at center ice. The other red dots (four of them) are next to the blue lines, and they're used if there's an infraction near them.

THE TEAM: PLAYER POSITIONS AND SHIFTS

As I mentioned in Chapter 1, most teams are made up of 16 or 17 players. There are usually nine forwards, six defense and one or two goalies. In a practice everyone is on the ice, but for games only six players per team are allowed on the ice at one time. Unless the coach is trying to take advantage of a delayed penalty or trying to tie the score very late in the game, the goaltender is always on the ice. If the coach pulls the goalie, another forward can be put in play.

The goaltender's job is to stop the other team from scoring. It's a tough position to play—so don't tolerate any players complaining about the quality of their team's goaltending. All the kids on a team, especially during the early years, should be given a chance to play goal. They'll know not to take it for granted.

The left- and right-wingers and the center make up the forwards. While the name of each position implies a specific area that the player must cover, it doesn't really work that way. The game is very fluid and players, especially forwards, will follow the play over the entire ice. The center typically chases the puck more and tries to "make the play"; that is, dump (or pass) the puck to a winger who is waiting just outside of a couple players who are battling for control of the puck. But often wingers do this. And defense, too.

Goal-scoring is the main task for forwards. They also need to be strong skaters who can carry the puck on a breakaway or rush back into their own zone to thwart the other team's chances of scoring. Often the same three forwards are played together. This is called a line. The players on a line get used to each other's style of play and can develop an uncanny ability of knowing where they are on the ice at all times. Sometimes a center can pass without looking and "know" the winger will be there to pick it up.

The defense players should be good at skating both backward and forward. They need to skate backward because often they're facing opposing players who are rushing in to try to score. On the other hand, when their own team is moving up the ice out of the defensive zone, the two defense players often shape the play as they wait for a forward to get into the open before passing the puck up to him or her. The best defense players thus keep a clear head when it comes to watching and understanding how a play is unfolding before sending the puck up the ice to a forward.

Individual players or whole lines (especially in the early years) come off the ice after a shift to let rested players take their place. This can often be frustrating for players (young and old) who always want to be on the ice where the action is. For Pre-Tyke, Tyke and Novice, a buzzer system is used to change players after two or three minutes (depending on your local association). When the buzzer sounds, all five skaters from each team go to their box and five fresh players come out for their shift. This helps keep everyone—parents and kids—calm about equal ice time. However, some kids are frustrated that they have to come off the ice when they feel they're just getting going. You may have to take some time to explain to your young player that everyone deserves an equal share of ice time and that the team does best when it has fresh players on the ice.

After two or three years of hockey, players start to change on the fly. This means a player comes to the team bench without waiting for a whistle, and a fresh skater takes his or her place. Changing on the fly usually starts at the Atom (11-year-old) level, although your league may do things differently. If your child is playing select or rep (all-star), players will start changing on the fly at an even younger age. But often the referee's whistle comes at a good point, and players will change then. Changing when the play is stopped is safer because there's less risk of being penalized for accidentally having too many players on the ice. The rule is that the player coming off the ice must be within 10 feet of the bench before the substitute player can go on. If the puck happens to come near the off-going player at this point, he or she must not make any attempt to play it.

A FEW BASIC RULES

Hockey's rules are laid out by the Canadian Hockey Association and USA Hockey. They're updated every year, but the main ones don't change very much. And, as I said above, your hockey association may have its own minor variations, intended to make things work smoothly in your particular situation.

Most things are pretty constant. For instance, there will be officials, known as referees, on the ice. They dress in elegant black pants and black-and-white striped shirts, usually topped off with a black helmet. Refs are whistle blowers: They do it to stop play whether for an off-side, a penalty or a goal. Their job—

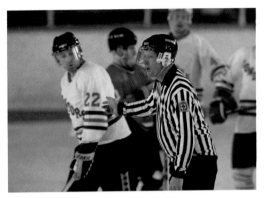

Referee in Action
The ref's job is to make sure the play is safe and fair.

and it's a tough one—is to make sure the game is played fairly and safely. (If you're interested in refereeing or learning about their training, take a look at Appendix 4.)

In the first couple of years of hockey, you'll usually see two officials, but as the players get bigger and the game gets faster, most leagues will have three. The head official is known as *the* referee and wears an orange or red armband. He or she calls penalties and signals when a goal is scored. The other two officials are known as linesmen and they are responsible for conducting the face-offs and making icing and off-side calls. (Be patient, I'll explain these somewhat arcane terms in the following pages.) Other game officials include the timekeeper, official scorer (or record keeper) and goal judges.

Off-side and Icing

New players and fans are often confused by two of the basic hockey rules—off-sides and icing. Luckily, if you keep hockey's objective in mind, they're not hard to understand.

The name of the game is to score. Now, one way of scoring would be to post a star player in the other team's end and wait for the rest of the team to dig out the puck and fire it down to where the star is waiting all alone. A good player, left

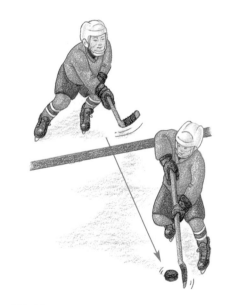

Off-side
The puck has to enter the zone before the advancing players. It cannot be passed ahead to a player already in the zone.

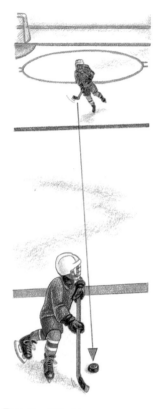

Two-line Off-side

The puck can't be passed over two lines to a teammate.

alone, can usually beat the goalie. So that would work, but it would be boring. The game is supposed to be about speed and skating and stick-handling, not rink-long passes.

The off-side rule is intended to avoid that sort of thing. What makes it complicated is that there are two kinds of off-sides.

The first off-side rule: If your child skates into the opposing team's zone *before* the puck enters the zone and then touches the puck, that's off-side. The linesman will whistle the play dead and the kids will start over, at a face-off outside the zone. (There are some complications, but that's basically it.) You can see how this would prevent the lone-player scenario I just sketched. To make it clear, let me add that your child is free to be the first on the team to cross into the offensive zone if he or she is carrying the puck, or if the puck is already across the blue line.

As I've said, the off-side is called when the offensive player already in the zone touches the puck that comes in after him or her. But in most leagues the offensive players can skate out of the zone again ("clearing the zone"), and no off-side will be called as long as they haven't touched the puck. If you see a linesman with one arm straight up, he or she has seen that a player is off-side but hasn't yet touched the puck. This "delayed off-side" is designed to keep the play going. If the player clears the zone by crossing back into the neutral zone, play continues and the linesman might further signal a "wash out" (no infraction) at this point with a sideways sweeping motion of both arms (as the umpire does in baseball).

One more thing: A goal can't be scored on a shot from outside the zone when an attacking player is off-side, even if the attacker hasn't touched the puck and the off-side hasn't been called yet. The linesman will blow the whistle as soon as there's an off-side shot on the net.

The second off-side rule: If the puck is shot from inside the defensive zone to a teammate who has both skates on the far side of the center red line, that's off-side. It's also known as a two-line pass because it crosses the blue line and the center red line. A two-line pass is legal in many kids' leagues (and in all college leagues), but it's banned in professional and junior ranks.

These rules can be hard for young children to understand. That's why many leagues enforce only the first rule, whose basic purpose is to prevent players from hanging around the other team's goal.

The other rule that causes confusion is icing. Here's the rule: If one team shoots the puck from its own side of the center red line across the other team's goal line, that's icing. The linesman's arm goes straight up, and he or she will stop play. The puck will be taken all the way back for a face-off at the other end of the rink. In kids' hockey, the whistle will go as soon as the puck crosses the goal line; in the pro ranks, a defending player must touch it first.

The icing rule prevents hockey from becoming Ping-Pong on ice. The game would become completely boring if a team could just throw the puck down the ice every time it got in trouble. That said, there is one situation in which icing is permitted (and you'll hear coaches and fans yelling "ice it!"), and that's when a team is short-handed (or down a player) because of a penalty. In this case, the short-handed team can (and should) shoot the puck to the other end of the rink. By the way, the team that isn't playing short-handed is said to be on a "power play" in this situation.

A complication: There's no icing if the linesman judges that a defending player could have got the puck before it crossed the goal line, but didn't try hard enough. There's also no icing if the goalie plays the puck before it crosses the red goal line.

ENFORCING THE RULES

The first consideration in youth hockey is safety. The refs can't afford to be lenient; they have to call what they see. If your child gets a penalty but isn't sure why, explain (or make sure the coach explains) the reason. Part of your job as a parent is making sure your child understands and respects the rules. Griping about bad calls and biased refereeing is no way to do that. I talk about this some more in Chapter 8.

Hockey has its idiosyncratic way of enforcing its rules. In football, an infraction brings a loss of yardage. In basketball, the victims of an infraction get a chance to score some points from the foul line. But in hockey, the rule-breaker is sent off the ice for a few minutes and the team has to struggle on short-handed. The short-handed team tries to "kill" the penalty (avoid being scored on); the other team has a "power play." Even if a team has several players penalized at once, it will still be allowed to put at least three skaters and the goalie on the ice.

Most penalties are so-called minors—the rule-breaker sits in the penalty box for two minutes but gets to come out sooner if the other team scores. Then there are

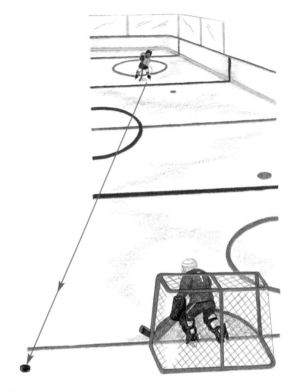

Icing
Players can't just dump the puck down the ice from behind the center line (unless his or her team is short-handed because of a penalty).

major penalties: five minutes, with no time off when the other team scores. The ref can also call a 10-minute misconduct, which banishes the player from the ice for (you guessed it) 10 minutes. In this case, though, the team is allowed to use a substitute. And finally, there's a game misconduct, which means the offender is gone for the rest of the game (although again the team does not have to play short-handed).

The only player who doesn't go into the penalty box is the goaltender. If the goalie gets a penalty, then another player serves the time.

(There are also match penalties and gross misconducts—punishments for more serious offenses, such as a deliberate attempt to injure a player—that usually result in suspension for several games or the remainder of the season. Fortunately, these serious offenses are very unusual in youth hockey.)

Then there's the penalty shot—the most exciting way of punishing an infraction. Penalty shots are called when an offensive player has a clear scoring chance and is fouled from behind. The ref can also call a penalty shot if a defensive player (not the goalie) grabs or falls on the puck inside the goal crease.

The penalty shot is one on one—a skater takes the puck at center ice and tries to score on the undefended goalie. But it's not as uneven as it might sound, especially if the goalie is hot and the attacker is not known for a scoring touch.

We'll get to the main penalties in a minute, but first a bit of strategy. Often, when there's a penalty, play stops right away. But sometimes, the referee just points an arm straight up to signal a penalty and lets the play go on. This is a "delayed penalty," and it happens when the team that was the victim of the infraction has the puck. After all, it would be unfair to deprive one team of a scoring chance because the other guys broke the rules. So the penalty is delayed until the bad guys touch the puck.

What this means is that the team with the puck has an advantage; the other guys can't score because the minute they touch the puck, play stops. So you'll sometimes see the ref with his arm in the air and the goalie skating frantically to the bench to be replaced by a sixth attacker. For a few seconds, one team will have a six-on-five advantage and, if they're good enough, they may even score. (If they do score, and the ref was intending to call a two-minute minor penalty, it will be waived. But a major penalty will still be called.)

THE MAIN PENALTIES

Here are the most common penalties, in alphabetical order. Except where it's noted otherwise, these are all two-minute minors.

In many rinks, the penalties are announced, but the ref will also give a hand signal that can be understood in the stands. If there are no announcements, of course, the hand signal is all you'll get. The diagrams will give you an idea of what to look for.

Boarding or Body-checking—if a player is checked into the boards in a violent manner, then the ref may call a boarding penalty. The ref's signal is the striking of a clenched fist into the open palm of the other hand in front of the chest. The same signal is used for body-checking in leagues where it isn't allowed. For instance, body-checking is not allowed in most youth leagues at or below the 11-year-old level. It's also forbidden in women's or girls' hockey, and some house-league associations ban body-checking at all levels.

Butt-ending—if a player jabs (or attempts to jab) another player with the shaft of the stick above the upper hand, a butt-ending penalty may be called. The ref holds one forearm over the other; the lower is moved back and forth, across the body.

Charging—if the player takes more than two steps or strides, or jumps into an opponent when body-checking, a charging infraction may be called. The referee signals by rotating clenched fists around each other in front of the chest. Since body-checking isn't allowed at the lower levels, you'll rarely see this called in the first few years.

Checking from behind—if a player pushes, body-checks or cross-checks an opponent from behind anywhere on the ice, a checking from behind penalty may be called. It's a game misconduct (ejection), coupled with a two-minute or five-minute penalty, depending on the severity of the offense. (A teammate will have to serve the two or five minutes if a game misconduct is called.) The ref's signal is a forward motion of both arms, with the palms of the hands opened and facing away from the body, fully extending from the chest at shoulder level.

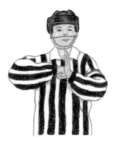

Penalty Signal
Boarding or
Body-checking

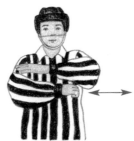

Penalty Signal
Butt-ending

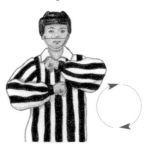

Penalty Signal
Charging

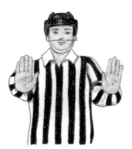

Penalty Signal
Checking from behind

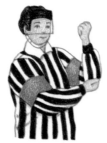

Penalty Signal
Cross-checking

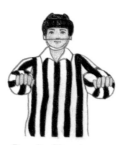

Penalty Signal
Elbowing

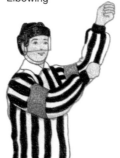

Penalty Signal
High-sticking

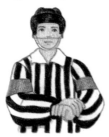

Penalty Signal
Holding

Checking from behind, even by accident, can cause serious injuries, particularly to the spinal cord. Players have to be in control of themselves, both physically (so as not to check from behind by accident) and emotionally (so as not to do it in the heat of the game). Part of your job as a parent is to make sure your child understands how serious checking from behind can be and how much you disapprove.

Cross-checking—using the shaft of the stick, held between the hands, to check an opponent at any height. The referee signals with a forward and backward motion of the arms with both fists clenched and about a foot apart. (The signal imitates the action of a cross-check.)

Elbowing—checking an opponent with the elbow. The referee signals by tapping either elbow with the opposite hand.

Fighting—this is pretty obvious. Players drop their gloves and flail away at each other. In the NHL, fighting is a five-minute penalty, but in youth hockey fighting is not tolerated. Fighters get a five-minute penalty and are ejected from the game. Unfortunately, a teammate has to sit in the penalty box for the full five minutes no matter how many goals the other team scores. There is no hand signal for fighting.

High-sticking—checking an opponent with the stick above the normal height of the shoulders, either purposely or accidentally. The referee holds both fists clenched, one immediately above the other at about forehead height. Some refs embellish the signal by making a slight chopping motion.

Holding—grabbing an opponent's body or stick with the hands. The referee clasps either wrist with the other hand in front of the chest.

Hooking—slowing an opponent down by hooking his stick on any part of the opponent's body or stick. The referee signals with a tugging motion with both arms.

Interference—impeding the progress of an opponent who doesn't have the puck. The referee crosses the arms in front of the chest. (No penalty, of course, for impeding the progress of a player who *does* have the puck, unless it's by high-sticking or holding or breaking some other rule.)

Roughing—if a player punches an opponent, that's roughing. The signal is a clenched fist and arm extended out to the front or side of the body. (If they both start throwing punches, of course, that's fighting.)

Slashing—hitting an opponent with the stick. The signal is a chopping motion with the edge of one hand across the opposite forearm.

Spearing—thrusting the blade of the stick at an opponent. Players are usually ejected from the game for spearing. The signal is a jabbing motion with both hands thrusting out in front of the body.

Tripping—using the stick or a body part to trip the puck carrier. This gets a little complicated, because if the checker touches the puck *before* tripping the opponent, there's no penalty. If there is a penalty, though, it's two minutes; the ref signals it by striking the leg with either hand below the knee, keeping both skates on the ice.

The ref can't see everything; his or her job is to make sure the action around the puck is fair and safe. From your vantage point in the stands, you may see things the ref can't see. It does no good at all to point these out to the ref; there will

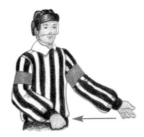

Penalty Signal
Hooking

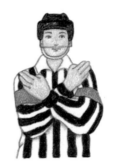

Penalty Signal
Interference

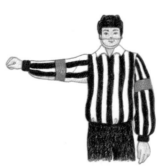

Penalty signal
Roughing

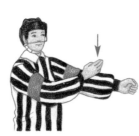

Penalty Signal
Slashing

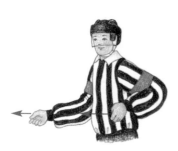

Penalty Signal
Spearing

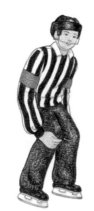

Penalty Signal
Tripping

never be a penalty called from the stands. And too much carping may give your child the impression that it's okay to bad-mouth the referees.

Another thing to remember is that not all penalties are "bad." Some penalties may actually result from a good play. For instance, a defense player may dive to bat away a puck from the other team's star scorer and thus incur a tripping penalty. If the trip took away a good scoring chance, it is often regarded as a fair trade, a "good" penalty.

Coaches say a penalty is "bad" when it is taken in the offensive zone. That's because the other team doesn't have a good scoring chance; they're in their own zone, sometimes without the puck. A penalty in this situation is usually seen as undisciplined.

Coaches also hate "retaliation" penalties. Sometimes, a player is tripped or hit, but the referee misses it. After all, the ref is busy following the play. But all too often, the ref notices the retaliatory slash or punch. Result: the "wrong" player gets sent off. Part of hockey is keeping a cool head at all times; parents can help by reminding players that the ref is human and makes mistakes. They can also help by reminding players that retaliation penalties are not only dumb—they're also not justifiable; a retaliating player is no better than the instigator. In fact, the best kind of retaliation is a goal or, even better, a win.

Obviously, I could say much more about how the game is played. But that would take a whole book, and there are other fish to fry. This brief overview should provide you with enough knowledge to be able to follow your child's games intelligently and to help him or her over some of the hurdles. As a side benefit, you may find you're being regarded as a bit of a hockey guru—all it takes is understanding the off-side and icing rules, and quietly muttering "off-side" or "icing" when the whistle blows.

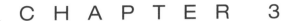

Playing the Game
The Basic Skills

As a parent, you can play an important role in the development of your child's hockey ability, even if you know little or nothing about the game. How? By understanding a few basics about the required skills and being able to transmit those to your child. As a coach for 10 years, I've learned that good hockey is based on skating, passing, puck control, shooting and checking. All the rest, as they say, is theory. In this chapter, you'll learn some of the essentials about those skills and I'll give you some hints on how you can help your son or daughter play better hockey.

SKATING

Skating is the bedrock. If you skate yourself, you can get your child started. In fact, you've probably already done that, and you're reading this book to learn how to take the next step into hockey.

But even if you can't skate, there's no reason why you can't go out on the ice in boots or running shoes and help your child learn the basics. Believe me, they're not going to go whizzing past you at this early stage. (If they do, of course, you are way ahead of the game.) On the other hand, if you really don't feel competent to teach your child to skate, there are other options. Almost every community has learn-to-skate programs, which are inexpensive and fun.

Because I'm a doctor, parents around the rink often ask how young is too young to learn to skate. My answer is: Once a child is walking and running comfortably, there is no reason not to try skating. I had my youngest son on skates at the age of one. He didn't skate, but he enjoyed just lying on the ice banging the puck around with his stick. By the time he was three, he was skating around like a pint-sized pro, stopping, turning, shooting and stick-handling. Not all children will do this—my son had older brothers to emulate, which certainly helps. And, of course, I'm a hockey enthusiast and love to teach the game. But you don't need to be an expert on hockey to get your child up on skates.

Here are a few tips to get kids on skates for the first time. Bear in mind that skating is a difficult skill to learn. The child will stand three inches taller than usual on two very narrow blades, and will try to move on a nearly frictionless surface. Luckily, kids don't have far to fall and their winter snowsuits make excellent padding.

Let's assume you have skates to fit your child. (See the sections on fitting and tying skates in Chapters 4 and 5.) Take an old piece of carpet and let the child walk around with the skates on just to get the feel of them. The skates should give enough support to keep the child's ankles from bending over. You might also buy a pair of junior double-wheel in-line skates (Fisher-Price makes one version). These just strap on to the feet, can be used indoors and out and—like walking around on the carpet—get the child used to the extra height and the narrow base of support.

Once your child is used to the feel of the skates, it's time to move to the ice. This is where the fun begins. Believe me, just getting kids to stand up on their own for the first time is a huge accomplishment.

The first thing a child—or any new skater—tries to do is walk or run on the skates. This is the first step to figuring out an actual skating stride, in which the pushing blade is at an angle to the gliding blade. Unfortunately, walking on skates doesn't work very well, because the ice is so darned slippery. This is where a small chair comes in handy.

Put the chair on the ice and let your child use it for support. (This will also save your back, because you won't be perpetually bent over.) The chair provides a broad base of support, and it won't take long—especially with your

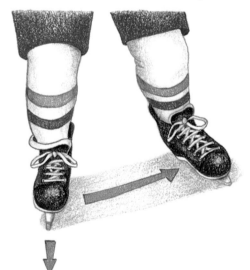

Starting the Stride
The rear skate pushes sideways and back on the ice. The front skate glides straight forward.

coaching—before the novice gets the idea of using one blade to push and the other to glide. Let the child use the chair as long as he or she likes; it will be discarded soon enough. One other advantage: The chair provides a great help when your child is trying to stand up after a fall and—believe me—there will be many tumbles and not a few tears. Make sure your little skater is well-padded (a snowsuit is usually enough), and there should be no problem.

This early stage can seem frustrating as your child tries to put several related skills together into one fluid motion. For example, you may find your child has a habit of pushing from only one leg. My eldest son did this when he was first learning. Don't worry—it will pass. In my experience—and I've just gone through it again, with my third son—learning to skate is very rewarding. Remember, to become a good skater, you have to spend a lot of time on the ice. The time your child spends on the ice during a regular game is probably less than 15 minutes—not nearly enough. Even a twice-a-week skating class is not really enough. So you have to find extra ice time. How? Try public skating. It makes a great family outing and exercises the same skills your child will need in hockey—skating in a straight line, stopping, and turning. Most community arenas offer convenient times.

As soon as kids have outgrown the chair, I like to give them a hockey stick. Again, this gives them extra support, like a third leg. In the beginning, kids really lean on the stick. Gradually, as they feel more comfortable, they straighten up and rely less and less on the stick for support. One lesson that will be helpful later is to keep two hands on the stick—something that comes naturally when using it for balance.

Balance, in fact, is an extremely important element when learning to skate. Even at the professional level, players continue to work on their balance—such as turning on one skate (to develop better control of their blade edges). For beginners, the stick jump is a good drill for developing balance while up and moving on skates. In this exercise, the kids skate toward a stick that's either lying on the ice or raised a few inches on pylons. When first starting out, children will likely glide toward the stick and then step over it. As they become more confident, they will go over the stick at greater speeds and without breaking their skating stride. The kids at my hockey school love this drill. (A more advanced version is to have kids do the stick jump while carrying the puck with their sticks. The puck is pushed under the raised stick while the players go over top in stride.)

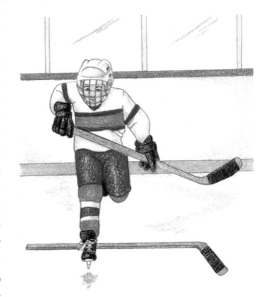

The Stick Jump
Drills like the stick jump are fun and develop balance.

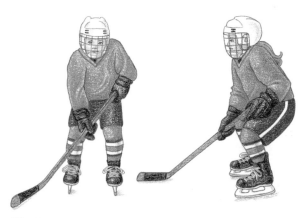

The Ready Position

Leaning forward with the knees bent gives the proper balance for skating. From this position the skater can move forward, backward and (with a little practice) even sideways.

You'll find that a few hours of shinny hockey—just fooling around with a puck and stick and a few friends—will do wonders for your child's skating. In many neighborhoods, kids now play street hockey on in-line skates, another fun activity that effectively increases their "ice" time. (Make sure they wear gloves and knee, wrist and elbow pads; a fall on in-line skates can cause some nasty scrapes.)

One simple tip that you can pass on to your child is to start in what I call the "ready" position. In this position, the skates are about shoulder-width apart, the knees are bent and the torso is leaning forward. From this position, your child can start skating in any direction without falling over backward.

A quick drill that you can use to help your child is the T-push. The child points one skate in the desired direction and puts the other one behind and crossways, forming a T. The knees stay bent and the body leans forward. Then the child pushes with the rear skate and glides on the other. The idea is that soon the child will be able to alternate pushes, first with one skate and then the other, and develop a complete skating stride.

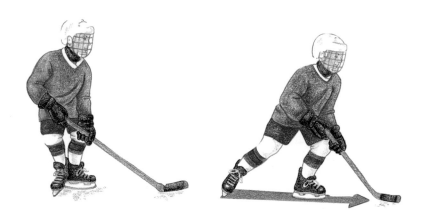

The T-push

The T-push is the start of a good stride. Push off by straightening the back leg as you glide on the front skate.

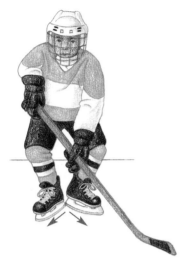

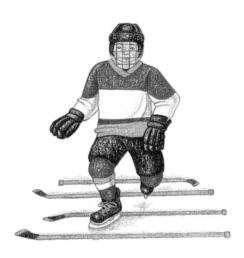

The V-start

The skates are pointed out like a V. The skater is in position to push off from either foot. Get up on your toes and take three quick strides.

Four-Stick Drill

Practice the V-start using four hockey sticks or old broom handles to jump or stride over. By having to take quick strides between the sticks, kids develop a faster, more powerful start. Be careful. If you glide, you'll hit the sticks.

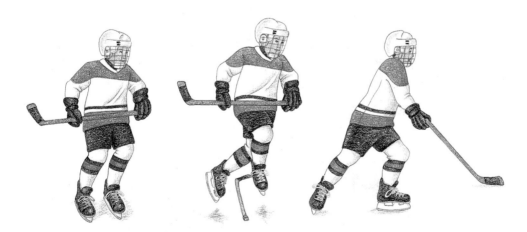

Crossover Start

Cross one skate over the other. This allows a player to start moving sideways. The first few strides are quick and choppy—then a regular stride can be taken. Practice this start by jumping over a stick. Also, remember to practice both left and right starts.

As your child's skating skills develop so will his or her ability to make a quick start. By becoming an efficient starter, a player can beat an opponent to a loose puck. The two basic starts are the V-start and the crossover start. Like all the skills I mention in the book, the best results come with lots of practice.

STOPPING

Once you've got the kids started, the time comes to teach them how to stop. Most kids learn quickly that they'll stop if they just glide into the boards and hang on. This, however, isn't the safest way. Instead of uncontrollably crashing into the boards, children are always better off learning how to stop wherever they need to.

The easiest stop to learn is the snowplow. In fact, the snowplow seems to come instinctively to kids when they try stopping themselves on skates. The child turns the skates toward each other, at about a 45 degree angle, and leans on the inside edge of the skate blade. If you're a skier, you're already familiar with the snowplow. On the ski hills, instructors sometimes tell kids to "make a pizza slice" with their skis. That's a good way of getting the idea across. What kid doesn't know about pizza?

You won't see NHL players using a snowplow stop, though. It really only works at the relatively slow speeds of 6- and 7-year-olds. Instead, more advanced players use the basic hockey stop.

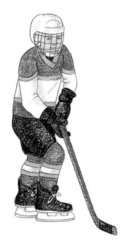
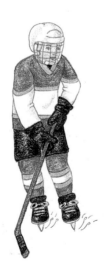
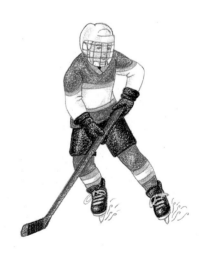

The Basic Stop

To stop, the blades of the skates dig into the ice.

In the basic stop, the skater shifts sideways quickly and slides to a halt with both blades across the line of travel. It's not the easiest skill to learn or to teach, because it requires both a sense of balance and a feel for the ice. If your child is having difficulty stopping, I would recommend three simple drills.

- Have him or her stand in the ready position, with the skates a little closer together than normal, and practice turning both left and right with the skates and body moving together. The idea is to become used to shifting one's weight while staying balanced.

- To help give your child a sense of how much pressure to apply to the skate edge, start from the ready position again and have the child slide one skate out to the side, scraping a bit of snow off the ice, and then return the skate to its initial position. Repeat the other way. The idea is to get a sense of how much pressure is needed to make the skate edges bite into the ice.

- Finally, have the child skate toward you, gliding in the ready position for the last 10 feet. Just as the child reaches you, he or she should try to stop by shifting the weight to one side and turning the skates. The idea here is that you're in a position to prevent a fall.

> **TIP** Try to make sure your child learns to stop, facing both ways.

TURNING

The first turn most kids learn is the simple glide. They stand on both skates and lean in the direction they want to go. Presto! They start to turn. One common mistake, by the way, is to drag the inside skate through the turn. As your child gains confidence and skill, tell him or her that both skates should be on the ice gliding forward. (In case you didn't know already, you'll likely need to remind your child more than once about that inside skate. Try not to be too critical, though. Some positive support and encouragement will go much further than sharp comments.)

Unfortunately, the gentle glide turn is often not useful in hockey because it's too slow. Instead, hockey players mostly use what are called—for reasons that will shortly become obvious—crossover turns. (There's also a type of turn called a power turn, but that's for when your child is a bit older.)

In the crossover turn, the outside leg crosses over the inside leg. (Who said hockey lingo is hard to understand?) The great thing about the crossover turn is that the skater can accelerate through a turn without losing any speed. But it is not an easy

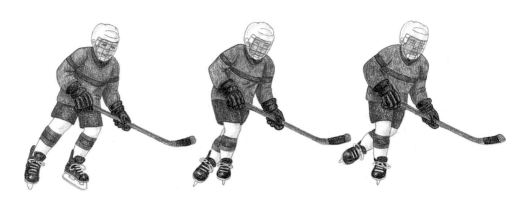

Crossover Turns

Crossover turns take practice. The player pushes from the inside skate while crossing over and forward with the outside skate. When the outside skate hits the ice and makes its stride, the inside skate is brought forward until it can start its push (or stride).

skill to master. Most kids will find it comes slowly, especially the little ones, whose legs are almost too short to cross over properly.

If you have access to ice, you might want to have your child practice skating in a figure-8 around two plastic pylons (or some other marker) placed about 10 feet apart—I think this drill is the cornerstone in developing a proficient skater. Another fun drill is to place some pylons around the ice to make a "slalom" course. Get the stopwatch out and time the kids. If there is a wide range of skill level, encourage the kids to focus on improving their own times rather than besting each other. Since most kids are better turning one way than the other, modify the course so the child has to turn more on his or her weak side.

> **TIP** Tell your child to twist the head and shoulders in the direction of the turn. If the skater is carrying a stick, it should be on the ice and also pointed in the direction of the turn.

SKATING BACKWARD

Backward skating is also a vital skill. The key here is posture. Tell your child to keep the knees and ankles bent, to lean forward a bit (but not too much), and to take the bottom hand off the stick. The head should be up (not looking down at the skates)—this way it

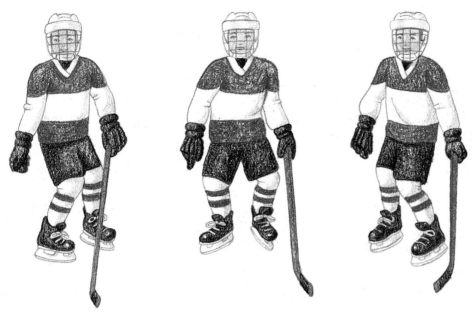

Backward Skating

Start by pushing from the front. The skate swivels out and cuts a C in the ice, while gliding backward on the other skate. Then the other skate takes over and cuts a C of its own. Try practicing the stride while hanging on to the boards.

can help swivel into turns much more easily. Then each skate blade, in turn, cuts a C-shape in the ice, moving from front to back. At first, this will seem awkward and difficult, but it will soon become second nature. (It's possible to practice by holding on to the boards or the bench and making C-cuts into the ice without moving.)

Over the long haul, the aim is to be able to skate backward as fast as forward. But that's not easy and certainly won't come immediately. So the earlier your child starts, the better.

> **TIP** Balance is key. If your child leans forward too much, he or she is likely to fall. That's why for skating backward there should be only one hand on the stick—using both hands makes the child lean forward too much. It's also important to keep the head up.

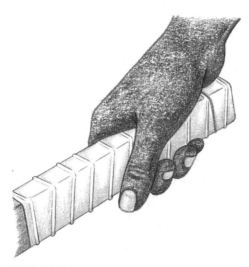

The Stick Grip
The thumbs should wrap around the shaft, as in a handshake.

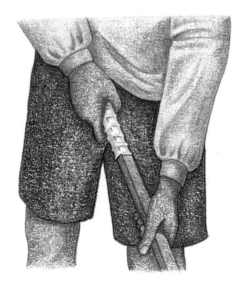

The Stick Grip (both hands)

HOLDING THE STICK

The proper grip is as important to a hockey player as it is to a golfer or a baseball player. I learned from one of the greats—Hockey Hall of Fame member Andy Bathgate, who coached me as a youngster. Encourage your child to hold the stick correctly from an early age. Believe me, as a parent or coach, you will have to remind your kid fairly often. I've sometimes been frustrated at my hockey school when I see kids who've been playing hockey for four or five years but who are still holding the stick incorrectly. Parents and coaches need to pay attention to this crucial element of play. At my school I always review the grip with the gloves off.

The top hand should go right at the end of the stick (or if your child uses a knob, just below the knob). The thumb goes behind the shaft and meets the tip of the forefinger, wrapping around. Believe it or not, the thumb generates a lot of the power in shooting and passing, so try to help your child get this right. The rest of the fingers curl around naturally.

If the top hand is correct, the thumb and index finger will form a **V**. The tip of the index finger wraps around to meet the thumb.

The bottom hand should grip the shaft in the same way, with the thumb and forefinger making a **V**-shape.

Many young players make the mistake of putting their thumbs on top of the shaft, which means their wrists and hands are in the wrong position. Consequently, their shots are also weaker.

I tell youngsters to think of shaking hands with the stick.

PASSING

At all levels of the game, passing is a difficult skill. Both ends of a pass—giving and taking—are skills you can help your child with. Like many skills in hockey, it's all technique and timing, which come only with practice. Encourage, but be patient.

The first thing is to make sure that the grip is correct. I like kids to have their gloves off when I teach passing, so I can watch their grip and wrist action.

To make a pass, the player has to perform three actions: wind-up, follow-through, and release.

- Wind-up: The child puts the stick in front of the puck and pulls it back a bit.

- Follow-through: The stick goes behind the puck and the child sweeps it forward, keeping the blade of the stick on the ice.

- Release: As the puck leaves the stick, the child rolls the wrists so that the tip of the stick-blade (the "toe" of the blade) is pointing at the intended receiver.

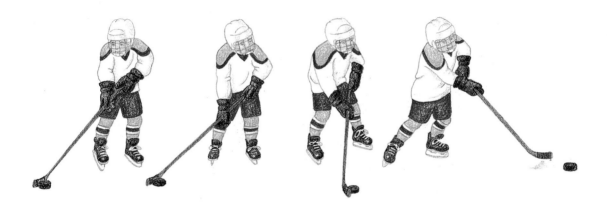

Passing: Wind-up, Follow-through, Release

Passing is much like sweeping a broom.

The whole motion is much like sweeping a broom, except for the snap of the wrists at the end. I teach kids to think that the toe of the blade acts as a guide for the pass, so it has to be pointed in the right direction.

A backhand pass is similar to a forehand pass, but done the other way. Have your child practice the backhand pass as much as the forehand. The tricky part of the backhand is that the shooter will want to face into the pass with his or her body. Most effective backhands are made when the player shoots almost perpendicular to the direction the body is facing. This is one reason why goalies fear the backhand most. There are fewer cues from the body as to which direction the shot will go.

To receive a pass you need to keep the stick on the ice. That may seem obvious, but it's not. Some kids just forget and others will say, "Oh, I can get my stick down in time." But they don't. This is the sort of thing that can give coaches fits. You can help by repeating the lesson: Keep your stick on the ice.

There are two reasons to keep the stick on the ice. One is to catch the puck, which travels (or should) along the ice for a pass. But perhaps more important is to give the passer a target, so he or she can make a good pass in the first place. I use the term "target" with my players to help the receiver keep in mind that the target, his or her stick, needs to be on the ice.

Here are three things you can show your child about actually taking the pass.

- Keep the blade at right angles to the line the puck is traveling on. Otherwise, the puck will glance off and the receiver will miss the pass.

- Cushion the puck as it arrives by moving the blade back just a fraction. This is a bit like "deadening" the baseball when bunting.

- The stick blade should be tilted slightly toward the puck, cupping it so that it can't jump over. (If the stick is gripped properly, the blade will tilt forward automatically.)

Practicing passing is extremely important. The skill can be mastered by practicing stationary passing with a partner. The kids stand about 10 or 15 feet apart, passing the puck back and forth just as in a simple game of catch. Later the kids can advance to moving passes. If the kids are ready for it, have them skate down the rink slowly in tandem, about 5 to 10 feet apart. They can pass the puck back and forth between them. Passing can also be practiced in the basement or the driveway with a foam puck or hockey ball.

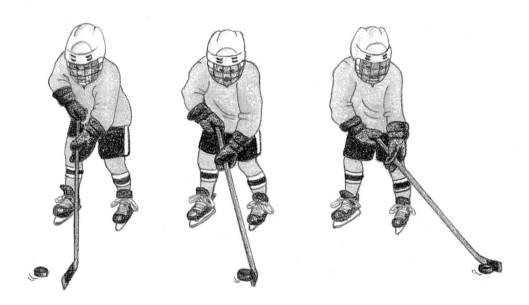

Receiving a Pass

The blade of the stick should be square to the pass and slightly tilted or cupped to prevent the puck from jumping over.

As you hang around the rink, perhaps watching some of the more advanced players, you'll hear lots of other passing terms. The snap pass is performed using a quick snap of the wrists. The flip pass (or saucer pass) involves flipping the puck over an obstacle, such as a defense player's stick. Obviously, this pass won't come until your child has mastered raising the puck. And then there are bank passes (using the boards like the cushion on a pool table), back passes (sending the puck backward to a player in a better position), drop passes (leaving the puck so another player can pick it up), and a host of others.

PUCK CONTROL

As you've probably figured out by now, the game of hockey is played with a puck. And you can't really play the game unless you can properly handle the puck, not just bat it around. In fact, the best piece of advice I ever heard came from Walter Gretzky, father of Wayne, who said kids should use a puck as much as possible in practice drills. He knew that old-time players didn't make it to the professional ranks unless they could stick-handle well. In fact, the earliest form of the game didn't permit forward passes, so the players *had* to stick-handle.

Today, stick-handling is almost a lost art. It's not really taught in organized hockey—and that's where your parental influence can come in. A backyard rink, if you have the space to build one, is an ideal place to learn stick-handling, simply because it is small. The confined space makes stick-handling the only way to play—outskating the others is moot on a 20-foot patch of ice.

If extra ice time is hard to get or even impossible, a child can learn a lot of skill and dexterity by practicing with a tennis or hockey ball outside or in the basement. If the child doesn't have anyone to play with, let him or her snap rebound shots with the ball against a basement wall or a solid fence. Even a sheet of "plastic ice" from your local hockey shop will let your child practice moving the puck back and forth, a basic motion which is the equivalent of dribbling in basketball. The idea is to feather the puck back and forth with a light touch, instead of a hard choppy action. Remember, stick-handling uses the wrists. The puck should be controlled with the toe and the middle of the blade, and the bottom hand should be fairly high on the stick—about a foot below the top hand.

When stick-handling the puck down the ice (like dribbling down the court in basketball), it's best for your child to keep the elbows from getting too bunched up against his or her sides. This way he or she will have an easier time rolling the wrists. The head should be kept up and the puck felt through the fingers.

As I said, the puck is best controlled with the middle and toe-area of the blade. At the heel it's more difficult and the player is apt to lose the puck. The lower hand for kids is optimally placed about 12 inches below the upper hand on the stick. Remember that stick-handling and puck control come from the wrists and fingers, but the child doesn't need to squeeze the shaft too hard. The feel is much like the way a baby grips your finger—there isn't much pressure, but just try pulling your finger away. Tell your child to grip the stick lightly and keep his or her elbows out. That will allow the wrists to roll and the fingers to feel the puck. Finally, of course, the head should be up.

All of this assumes, by the way, that the stick is sized correctly (see Chapter 4). The stick needs to be short enough so that when making a tight turn away from the shooting side (if the player shoots left and is turning a fast right), he or she can move the arms and hands across the front of the body while keeping the stick blade flat on the ice. If the stick is too long, the blade must be lifted off the ice for tight turns, and that can mean missed passing and scoring opportunities.

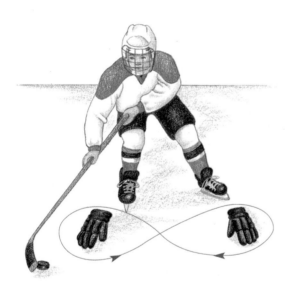

Stationary Stick-handling Practice

One of the undertaught skills in kids' hockey, stick-handling can be practiced at home (with a tennis ball) or on the ice. Also, with the gloves off you can see the player's grip.

At my hockey school, I have the kids do the figure-8 drill (the same as in the skating and turning sections of this chapter), but with a puck. It's a great way to improve puck control. So is a "slalom." I have the kids just put their gloves on the ice a few feet apart and move the puck around these "obstacles." All of this prepares the young player for more advanced skills that he or she will pick up as the years go by, such as deking and faking opposing players or sneaking a quick shot around a goalie.

Remember that you don't need a sheet of ice to practice stick-handling. A piece of inexpensive plastic ice is available at sporting goods shops. Stick-handling can be practiced on this "ice" in the driveway or in the basement. As I already mentioned, even stick-handling a tennis or hockey ball or a foam puck on a smooth cement surface will help develop coordination and skill in the off-season.

SHOOTING AND SCORING GOALS

I believe that goal-scoring can be taught to children. It may seem obvious, but most goals are scored from about 10 feet in front of the net with a low shot. This area is the shooting zone, otherwise known as the slot. One tip you can give your child (assuming he or she is playing forward) is, "Go to the slot."

Once in the slot, of course, your child is going to have to shoot the puck—and this takes two things: knowing how to shoot, and knowing where to shoot.

You'll sometimes hear people talk about scoring on the "five-hole." This is shorthand. There are five places where the puck reasonably might go in the net, assuming the goalie is in position: in the four corners or between the goalie's legs. The five-hole is the area between the goalie's legs. Obviously, if the goalie has his or her legs together, the five-hole is closed off and there's no sense shooting there.

I like to tell kids to shoot for the corners, especially the bottom corner on the goalie's stick side, which is often a weak area. A so-called stand-up goaltender (who tends to remain upright) often has trouble covering this spot. In contrast, a butterfly goalie (who goes down with pads spread out like a butterfly's wings) will cover the bottom corners well, but often leave open the five-hole and upper corners.

Shooting takes practice. Lots and lots of practice. Luckily, it's one of the few hockey skills that doesn't require ice time. Pick up a hockey net (at a sporting goods store or a garage sale) and a sheet of plastic ice. Get some pucks, and you have everything you need for your child to practice shooting year-round. If you put a chair in front of the net, or dress up a dummy as a goalie, you'll make it more challenging (and fun) for your child. Practicing shooting is important because beginning players may get only one or two scoring opportunities in a game.

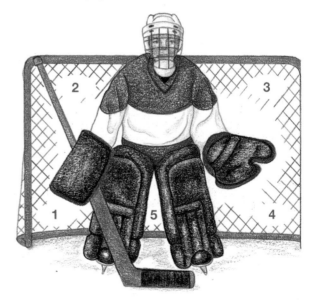

The Five Holes

If the goalie is in position, there are five areas to shoot at.

As you hang around the rink, you'll hear terms like wrist shot or snap shot. Hockey shots can be lumped into five categories—the wrist, snap, flip, slap and backhand shots—but the basic principles are the same for all of them. To tell you what makes a truly great shooter—a Paul Kariya or a Wayne Gretzky—would take another book. But there are some tips you can pass on.

Ask your child to try to make sure the puck is between the middle of the blade and the toe. That's where he or she will have the most control and the most power. If the puck is near the heel of the blade, the shot won't work.

All kids want to develop a huge slap shot. There's something very satisfying about taking that big wind-up and really bashing the puck. But as a parent, you should encourage the wrist shot and the backhand shot first. As I said earlier, a good backhand especially is hard for goalies to handle. A slap shot is harder to control and may even be forbidden by your child's league.

The wrist shot and the backhand shot are much like the forward and backhand pass—there's a wind-up, a follow-through and a release, in which the wrists roll over. A key part of the shot is the transfer of weight from the back skate to the front, as the shot is released. Much of the power in a shot comes from the legs, not the wrists and arms. Remember, the child needs to be holding the stick correctly for these shots to work.

For my money, the biggest mistake kids make is not rolling their wrists over as they release the puck. If your child is having trouble shooting well, that could be the problem. The result is a weak shot that is easily blocked.

Almost any goalie will tell you that a backhand is the most difficult shot to stop, because it's hard to judge its direction as it comes off the blade. So developing a good backhand can be a real asset.

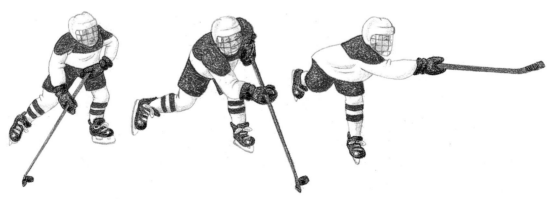

The Wrist Shot

Much of the wrist shot's power comes from the legs. The shooter's weight transfers from the back leg to the front. Make sure the grip is correct and the hands are properly placed on the stick. The wrists roll over as the puck is released.

CHECKING

Hockey in its simplest form is a game of many small one-on-one battles for control of the puck. The team that wins most of these little checking battles wins the game. Checking just means trying to get the puck away from another player or covering an opponent. It's a central part of the game.

A good checking practice is the puck race. Two kids pair off at one end of the rink and race for the same puck at center ice. This type of drill teaches the player what I call contact confidence (see the following section—Body Contact and Checking—for more on this). In the puck race, the two players bump against each other as they scramble for the puck, and it's the player who can best keep the stick on the ice (to grab the puck) and use the body (to keep on track for the puck) who usually ends up with the puck. It's a fun drill for the kids, especially if the coach makes an effort to match the players evenly.

Stick-checking comes in several forms. There's the stick-lift, in which the defensive player lifts the puck-carrier's stick to try to get the puck away. And there's the hook-check, where the defender tries to hook the puck off the other player's stick. The defender can poke the puck away, using a quick, well-timed "poke-check." Or the player can just press down on the opponent's stick, preventing him or her from stick-handling, passing, shooting or making a puck grab.

If you hang around any hockey rink, you'll hear the terms forechecking and backchecking. Forechecking means checking in the other team's zone, hoping to regain possession of the puck or to slow the opposition's advance. Backchecking means checking in the neutral or defensive zone, hoping to prevent a scoring opportunity. It's called backchecking because it's usually done by the forwards, who must come back into their own zone to do it. A lazy forward, who hangs around up the ice while the opposition is mounting an attack, will often draw the scorn of teammates and spectators alike.

BODY CONTACT AND CHECKING

There's a difference between checking and body-checking. When one team has the puck, the other team must check to try to regain possession. Using the stick to lift an opponent's stick or bat the puck away is one way of trying to get the puck (I talked about that in the previous section). Body-checking—using the body to knock an opponent off the puck—is another way. For the most part, body-checking (as opposed to body contact) is not allowed in kids' hockey. In some hockey associations it's allowed once the players are 12. It's never allowed in girls' hockey, and some mixed or boys' house leagues may ban it at all levels.

In fact, for the most part, body-checking is confined to rep (all-star) or select programs. If you want to avoid body-checking, there's a simple answer: Keep your child out of rep and select hockey. Do not let him or her try out for those teams.

As I said, in all likelihood your child is not going to be involved in full-contact hockey for several years, if at all. But hockey is a fast-paced sport, played in a confined area, and body contact—not deliberate body-checking—is unavoidable. If nothing else, players will occasionally run into each other. This is why children still need to be well protected even though no body-checking is allowed.

At my hockey school and when I'm coaching, I like to tell kids to be extra aware of themselves and their opponents when they're within a couple of feet of the boards. This is the danger zone. Out in the middle of the ice, falling or being knocked down is no problem, although it may hurt for a moment or so. But in the danger zone, even a simple but awkward fall can be hazardous. Here are some things you can teach your child:

- Keep the head up at all times.

- Keep the stick down.

- Know where your opponents are.

- Always go to the boards at an angle, not straight on. Going straight in after a puck can result in pitch-forking on the stick and being catapulted head-first.

- Get up against the boards when fighting for the puck.

- Keep the skates parallel to the boards.

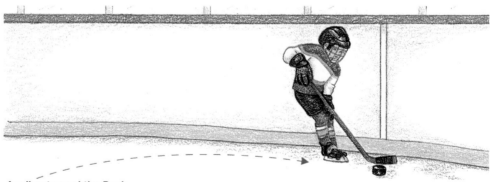

Angling toward the Puck

Always keep the skates at an angle to the boards. *Never* skate straight toward the boards to pick up a puck.

A player whose head is down and whose skates are perpendicular to the boards is asking for trouble—trouble that at its worst can be a serious spinal injury. And it can happen even if there's no body-checking allowed. In all my years of coaching and teaching I've never seen this happen. But I've heard about it. So teach the kids to play smart. Every child player needs to know: *Do not put yourself in a position where you can be hit from behind, even accidentally, and driven into the boards head-first.* (Former NHL player Mike Bossy has an excellent video on this; see Appendix 5.)

At my hockey school, we teach contact confidence. I think it's important because even if body-checking isn't allowed in your child's league, body contact (intentional or not) is inevitable in any game. A fun drill for very young kids is to have them skate straight at the coach, who holds a padded object (like the base-bag used in baseball) in front of his or her chest. The skater drives his or her shoulder into the bag as if giving an actual body-check. Another fun drill is to have the kids bump shoulder to shoulder as they slowly skate around the rink. Both these drills help with balance, and the kids also learn that checking doesn't hurt if they're in proper position—stick down, head up, knees flexed and the skates at least shoulder width apart. Not all hockey schools do this, but I think it's a must.

When I was a young player, we didn't have full face shields. I well remember the pain of getting a puck or stick in the face or having my nose rubbed along the boards. But I quickly learned to keep my head up and my stick on the ice. I learned to look before I went into the corner and always to angle toward the puck. Happily, helmets and face shields have virtually eliminated eye and face injuries in today's game. But the byproduct of that has often been a lack of respect for other players and more carelessness in the use of the stick and the body.

With all the equipment and high safety standards of today, kids look like modern-day gladiators when they're dressed to play. On top of that, they often feel invincible. Don't let yourself or your child be deceived into thinking that the equipment—no matter how expensive it is—will completely make up for carelessness on the ice. Teach them ice smarts: Head up. Stick down. And *never* skate straight toward the boards.

Remember, even when body-checking is not allowed, our job as parents is to emphasize safe (and fair) play.

SUMMING UP

The basic skills in hockey are not so basic. They can be challenging and time-consuming to master. But practicing these skills will immensely improve your child's hockey experience. The skills should be taught in a friendly atmosphere, always with an explanation about why the skill is important and when it is used in a game. If you're watching a game on television or in the rink, try pointing out to your child the different skills the players are using. But for now, as your child begins his or her hockey career, remember that hockey's basics take years to learn properly. Focus on what your child does right. Give tips and coaching sparingly, and never too much at one time. Encourage, encourage, encourage.

CHAPTER 4

The Equipment
What Your Child Needs

COST, SAFETY AND USED EQUIPMENT

The first thing new hockey parents ask is, How much does equipment cost? And the second thing they ask is, How do I know I've got the right stuff? In this chapter and the next, I'll try to answer those questions, giving you tips on how to keep the cost down and how to make sure your child's equipment does its job.

One important tip: Proper fit is vital, so make sure your child is with you when you buy equipment. You don't want to guess when it comes to your child's safety or comfort.

The first thing to remember when you're contemplating equipment is that hockey is a game played at high speed, at least in principle. In fact, for young kids, it tends to resemble a pack of puppies wrestling on a shiny kitchen floor, falling down, getting up, making a great effort and getting nowhere very fast. So you might think that getting good equipment and making sure it fits is less important in the first years than it will be later, when speed begins to play a part. Nothing could be further from the truth. Accidents can happen at any age. And good equipment can keep them from being serious. So make sure you get equipment that will keep your child safe.

Does that mean you have to spend an arm and a leg? No. In most cities and towns, there are skate and equipment exchanges where you can get perfectly good used equipment for much less than new. A good rule of thumb when buying used equipment is to pay about half the retail price if the gear is in good shape. If it's more than that you may want to shop around a little longer. Your community center or local hockey association may run an annual sale of outgrown equipment. And there are businesses that specialize in used equipment. You need to know two things to use these outlets with confidence: how to recognize good equipment, and how to make sure it fits. When I discuss individual pieces of equipment later in this chapter, I offer more pointers about buying used.

GIRLS' EQUIPMENT

Let me say a few words about girls' hockey equipment. The growth of women's hockey has led equipment manufacturers to notice that women are built differently than men. As a result, specialized equipment designed to fit the mature female anatomy is now available. Typically, the equipment is lighter and smaller, as well as being shaped differently. For older girls and women, the pants are shorter and slimmer at the waist. Shoulder pads are designed to support and protect the breasts. Gloves for women are narrower and have shorter fingers. However, instead of buying specialized equipment, many women and older girls simply buy boys' or men's equipment of the appropriate size.

In fact, for a young girl, the equipment can be the same as for her brother. After all, 7-year-olds have pretty much the same build whether they are girls or boys. For most readers of this book, specialized equipment is several years in the future. This simplifies finding gear, since at hockey exchanges and garage sales you are likely to see much less stuff for girls.

The exception of course is the jockstrap, which protects the genitals from stray pucks and sticks. For obvious reasons, girls don't need the roomier protective cup for boys. But they do need protection and they get it with the rather cutely named jillstrap (it's more prosaically called a pelvic protector). These are widely available, and I discuss them along with jockstraps later in this chapter.

THE HELMET

I strongly urge you to buy a new helmet. The reason is simple—you don't know the history of a used one. Has it been carefully treated? Has it been battered around? Is the padding still in good shape? Are there microscopic cracks in the plastic that could cause it to fail when it's most needed? Is it too old to be safe?

Manufacturers recommend that helmets should be replaced after five years. Why? Because they weren't designed to last forever. So don't take a chance. A top-line helmet, featuring what's called a "dual-density foam" lining, will cost about half

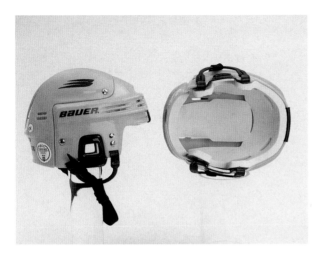
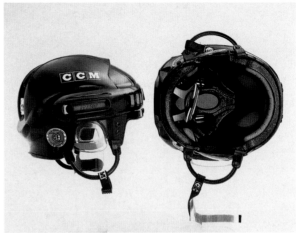

Standard and Top-line Helmet
Helmets have different types of linings, which accounts for much of the difference in price. The top-line model on the right costs almost twice as much as the one on the left. Either will do the job fine.

again or even twice as much as a standard model. For most children, a standard helmet—which used to be the state of the art, of course—is just fine. You'll also need a facemask, which will up the ante.

One thing to note—the helmet is designed to protect the brain and skull from injury. It will *not* prevent neck injuries. That's one reason coaches tell kids to keep their heads up—so they won't have collisions, with the boards or with other players, that could injure their necks.

Now to the nitty-gritty.

Helmets come in different colors, and some hockey associations prefer that kids have a specific color. If that's an issue, it may cut down on your choice of model and make. Usually, though, either white or black will be acceptable. If your hockey association requires a red helmet, though, don't be tempted to cheat by buying a white one and a can of red spray paint. Repainting a helmet or applying decals will weaken the shell and void the warranty. (You can, however, put your child's number on the back with stickers available at any sporting goods store.)

Helmets also come in size ranges and must be adjusted to fit your child's head. If you're in luck, the folks at the equipment store will know what they're doing and you can sit back and watch as junior gets the helmet custom-fitted. If you're not in luck, you'll have to do it yourself.

Here's how to do it. You'll probably need a screwdriver, although some of the newest models have a tool-less adjustment feature. Loosen the adjustment screws and pull the helmet open as far as possible. (The pieces will slide to the front and back.)

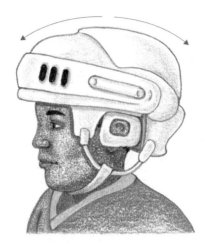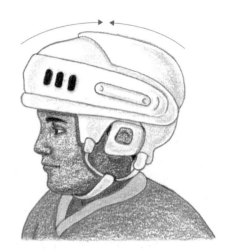

Fitting the Helmet

Loosen the adjustment screws and pull the helmet open as far as possible. (The pieces will slide to the front and back.) Once loosened, the helmet can be fitted properly to your child's head.

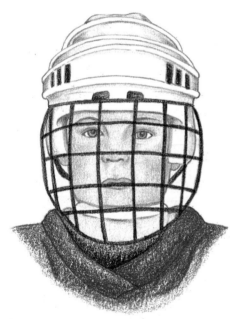

Properly Fitted Helmet (and Facemask)

The rim of the helmet should be a finger's width above the eyebrows.

Put it on the child's head, with the front rim a finger's width above the eyebrows. Slowly tighten the helmet until it fits snugly. Then tighten the adjustment screws again. The helmet should not slip back and forth; if it does, it's too loose. At the same time, your child shouldn't be getting headaches; that's a sign the helmet is too tight. Don't let your child wear the helmet so that it rides high on the forehead; it won't provide adequate protection.

The ear protectors, by the way, are removable. But leave them on. They are there to protect the ear from a high stick or a puck.

Lastly, let's discuss the chin strap. If you've ever watched an NHL game, you may have noticed the pros tend to wear their chin straps dangling down about four inches off the chin. Not surprisingly, the helmet goes flying off in the wake of a collision or a fall. It's simple: If the chin strap is not done up correctly, the helmet can't function properly. A good rule of thumb is you should be able to get a finger between the chin strap and the chin.

There are fewer varieties of helmets than there are, for instance, skates, but the choice is still large. Don't be intimidated. As I mentioned, the main difference between a manufacturer's top-line helmet and a cheaper model will usually be in the lining, which is designed to absorb the force of an impact. A top-line model will have a better liner system, as well as more bells and whistles—such as the tool-less adjustment system. But for most kids, a standard helmet will provide all the protection they need. I hesitate to recommend models or manufacturers because a helmet's fit depends so much on the shape of your child's head.

THE FACEMASK

For obvious reasons, a facemask of some sort is mandatory in children's hockey, both in the United States and Canada. Facemasks come in three basic types: a wire cage, a clear plastic shield and a combination cage-plastic shield. Each does the job, but each also has its pros and cons. It's a matter of taste which your child prefers. For instance, the wire cage is simple and requires no maintenance, but some kids find the bars in their peripheral vision are a distraction. The clear shield solves that problem, but can fog up because it has less ventilation than the cage. It also has to be protected to avoid scratches.

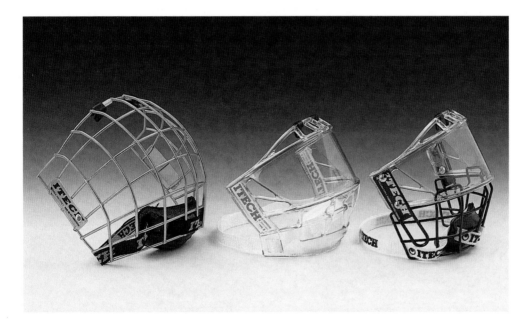

Facemasks

From left to right: The wire mask, the full visor and the combination mask. The standard wire cage is the most economical and will last the longest.

The fogging issue—which also applies to the combination mask, although not as much—can be combated with an antifog solution, which is rubbed on the plastic before a game. And many plastic shields now come with an antifog coating, which somewhat alleviates the problem.

However, unlike the wire cage, the plastic is susceptible to scratches. If you decide to go the plastic shield route, make sure you have a cloth pouch that fits over the mask whenever it is in the equipment bag. But no matter how careful you are, the mask will get scratched. Because of that, manufacturers recommend plastic shields be replaced every year (and I agree with them). It's a good idea to keep some visor cleaner in the hockey bag.

A wire cage (the cheapest of the three varieties), on the other hand, will last for years—as long as it isn't damaged or broken. (A word of warning: Never cut any of the wires to improve your child's view. You'll weaken the cage and compromise safety. You'll also void the warranty.) The cages come in different colors. Some kids find that a black cage impairs their vision less than a white one.

The simplest way to buy a facemask is to get one that's already mated to a helmet and sold as a unit. But if that's not possible for some reason, be aware that not all masks fit all helmets. The best plan is to have the helmet with you when you buy the mask. That way, you're in no danger of getting a mismatch.

You may see a number from one to six on the side of the mask. This is the Canadian Standards Association rating, which defines who should wear the mask. So, for instance, a type-three mask is for goaltenders. If your child isn't planning on playing goal, you should be looking for either a one or a two, depending on your kid's age. A type-one mask is for non-goalies older than 10, while a two is for non-goalies younger than 10.

> **TIP** The mask will loosen from time to time, so keep a screwdriver handy. It's also not a bad idea to buy some extra screws and keep them in the child's hockey bag.

THE MOUTH GUARD

Internal mouth guards have become the latest piece of protective equipment for children, but I have to confess, as a doctor and as a hockey coach, I have some concerns about them.

An internal mouth guard is a plastic device that fits over the top teeth. The idea is to prevent the teeth from slamming together in a collision and either breaking the teeth or perhaps biting off a piece of tongue. They certainly can help prevent such injuries. But there's a debate in the medical and dental communities: Do they also protect against concussion or head injuries if there's a blow to the jaw? If you're really concerned about your child's teeth, talk to your dentist.

As with anything, the more you pay, the better the product. A mouth guard custom-fitted in a dentist's office will be made of better materials and be more comfortable to wear. I prefer the custom-fitted mouth guards—if you want your child to use one—but they are costly. You could easily spend one or two hundred dollars on a custom-fitted mouth guard and, of course, it will have to be replaced every year.

Conversely, the mouth guards you fit yourself won't be as good, but they'll be a lot cheaper. Any sporting goods store will have a selection of mouth guards. You take them home, drop them into boiling water to soften them, and (after they've cooled a bit) press them onto your child's top teeth. To make the mouth guard fit, you'll probably have to cut the ends off with scissors. Some mouth guards attach to the mask with a strap so are harder to lose, but they can be easily removed.

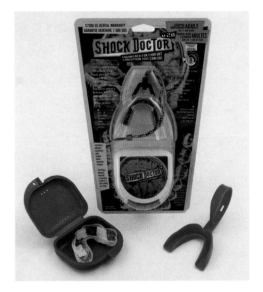

Mouth Guards

Your dentist can make a custom mouth guard for your child like the one on the left. Sporting goods stores will have a selection of inexpensive do-it-yourself mouth guards like the two on the right.

In the United States mouth guards are mandatory from Peewee on up (they must be colored and attached to the facemask so the referee can be sure it's being worn). For children's hockey, mouth guards are not mandatory in Canada. When I played university hockey, I wore an internal mouth guard. It was mandatory because the only other face protection we wore was a plastic half-visor to protect the eyes. So as a player I have some experience with mouth guards, and I'm still not sure they're a good idea.

Personally, I worry about the effect of mouth guards on the game. To my mind, there's no doubt a mouth guard will interfere with communication on the ice—things like calling for a pass or warning a teammate of an approaching checker. Mouth guards also reduce the size of the mouth cavity and can interfere with breathing. And they're easily misplaced: Even experienced players, like the teenage Juniors I work with, lose their mouth guards regularly.

But the main reason I don't like mouth guards is this: They're another piece of equipment we put on our kids to make them feel invincible. Let's face it, if your child is wearing a full mask, the chances of a significant dental injury are low. And we are not seeing large numbers of concussions in young hockey players. What we are seeing is young children developing bad habits that they carry with them to higher levels—Bantam, Midget and Junior. The answer to injuries at those levels is not more equipment at all levels, but better education at the lowest levels. Children must learn how to treat other players with respect, the rules must be enforced, and coaches and parents must understand how to make the game safe, as well as fun.

THE SKATES

If I could give one piece of advice to the hockey parent who is trying to figure out what equipment warrants greater expense than the rest, it is this: Put your money in skates. Hockey stores have an overwhelming selection of skates; the prices are even more overwhelming. But the investment is worth it. A good pair of skates, properly fitted, will make all the difference in your child's enjoyment of the game.

Still, making the right choice isn't easy. As a guideline, the midprice skate from any of the major manufacturers will do just fine. I encourage you to stick with the major manufacturers for a reason. Making a good skate takes plenty of experience, and newcomers to the field may not immediately reach the same level of quality.

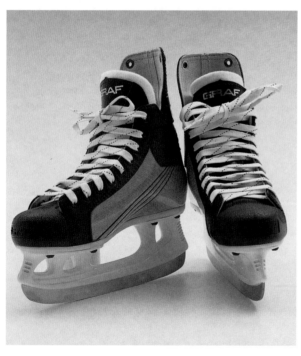

Skates
Put your money in skates. I think parents' hockey budget is best spent on a good pair of skates.

Widget Running Shoes *may* make a fine skate, but I'd hedge my bets and go with CCM or Bauer or one of the other long-time skate makers. A used pair, of course, would be significantly cheaper. I talk more about buying used skates at the end of this section.

Skate sizes are usually one lower than the shoe size. Youth sizes range from 8 to 13, and junior sizes from 1 to 6. Senior sizes are from 6 up. But, as with shoes, CCM's size 10 may not be exactly as big as Bauer's size 10, so you have to watch out for that.

I suggest buying skates at a hockey store or a sporting goods store that's strong in hockey. The salespeople there will usually have some expertise and be able to discuss the pros and cons of the different models. If you try to buy skates at a hardware store, on the other hand, you're going to be on your own. That's fine if you know exactly what you want, but it could be trouble otherwise.

Kids aren't great at saying how things fit, and because skates have a rigid toe, it's hard to tell from the outside. Here's a simple test: Loosen the laces of the skate and have the child push his or her toes to the front end. If you can get a finger behind the heel, the skate fits.

As with all equipment, of course, you need the child there. Don't buy a size 8 just because Johnny or Josie wore a size 7 last year. Also, when you go to buy skates, make sure that your child brings the type of sock he or she normally likes to wear inside the skates. (Thin cotton socks are best.) Some players—my eldest son among them—prefer bare feet in their skates. If the skate fits, with little or no movement of the foot, blisters won't be a problem.

In general, correctly sized skates will last one season. If they last for two, they were too big the first year. In fact, if your child is going through a growth spurt, you may find a new pair of skates is needed halfway through the season. This expense will seem less extravagant if there's a younger sibling or another relative or friend to pass the old skates on to.

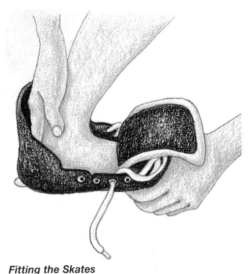

Fitting the Skates

If you can get a finger behind the heel, there's usually enough room for a season's growth but the skate otherwise fits snugly.

The skate has three main parts: the boot, the blade-holder and the blade. Skates used to have leather boots, steel blades and steel blade-holders, all of which made the skate extremely heavy. Now the boots are made of a variety of flexible synthetics, the blade-holders are strong but lightweight plastic, and only the blades are steel. The result is that modern skates are light and comfortable.

If you're buying used skates, there are some things to watch out for:

- Are there cracks in the blade-holder? If there are, take a pass.

- Are all the rivets in place?

- How much blade is left? If you notice that there's almost no blade showing outside the blade-holder, take a pass. It probably means they've been traded in several times.

- Are there soft spots in the reinforced toe? If so, definitely take a pass.

- Are the blades showing rust? If they are, they're not stainless steel. Take a pass. (If you're buying new skates, you can go with cheaper carbon steel blades, because you'll be taking care of them and preventing rust.)

- Squeeze the boot at the ankle. There should be some resistance. If there isn't, don't buy.

- And lastly, if you are buying used, you may come across all-plastic skates of the sort that were quite popular in the 1980s. Avoid these. Newer skates have plenty of ankle support and will get your child accustomed to the type of skate he or she will most likely wear over the years.

Breaking in Skates

New skates are stiff and have to be broken in—something I always hated. Luckily, there are some tricks to make it easier. Before I continue, though, I urge you *not* to send your child to hockey school or team tryouts in brand-new skates. It's a recipe for sore feet.

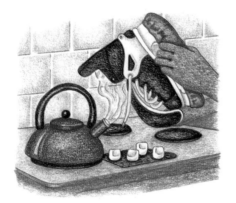

Breaking in Skates
Breaking in new skates will go more quickly if you use Hamlin (Hammer) Smith's kettle trick.

One way to break skates in is to wear them around the house—with the skate guards on, of course. Or pack the child up and go pleasure skating a few times.

As well, some sporting goods stores will have skate ovens—which are, as the name implies, small ovens that warm skates. The child puts a foot in the warmed skate and it molds to fit. If skate ovens aren't an option, you can try another trick at home. Take the liners out of the skates. Boil some water in a kettle, place the skate boot over the steam for about five or ten minutes, then put the liner back in and have the child put the skate on. It will begin to mold to the foot. (I'm obliged to Hamlin Smith, the athletic trainer for the Brampton Battalion and the 1999 Team Canada Junior team, for this idea.)

Tying the Skates

Every weekend, in every hockey arena in the world, parents hear the clarion call: "Will you tie my skates?" And mom or dad grabs a foot and tries to jam it into a skate that just doesn't want to go on. I sigh every time I see parents wrestle with their kids' skates. It's so easy.

Take the laces out of the top three or four eyelets and pull the tongue forward. The foot will slip in without much effort at all. Of course you have to relace the boot, but the saving in time and frustration is worth it. Before tying the skate up completely, though, have the child bang the heel on the ground to get the foot in the back of the boot. And as you tie it up, keep the skate low to or even on the floor, so the foot won't slip forward again.

Some kids don't like the lace through the top eyelet because they think it interferes with ankle movement. It's okay to leave the top eyelet unused. If you do use it, though, make sure the lacing up top is not too tight or the laces will dig into the child's ankle.

Some people buy long laces and then wrap the ends of the laces around the ankle before making a knot. I don't like doing this. In my view, it interferes with movement. If the ends of the laces are too long, buy smaller laces. (Once you know the right lace size (in inches), write it inside the skate boot so you won't forget.)

And remember: Laces have to be replaced from time to time. Replace them if they become frayed at the end. And replace them a couple of times a year anyway, because they do lose their strength and holding ability. It's a good idea to keep an extra set in the hockey bag.

It's a milestone when kids can do up their own skates. Personally, with three kids, I dream of that day.

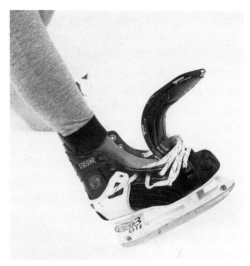

Tying the Skates
It's easy to get your kid's skates on—if they're loosened properly.

Skate Sharpening

The first thing to do with new skates is to get them sharpened. Most arenas have a pro shop, with an attendant whose main job is to sharpen skates. As well, most hockey equipment stores will have a skate sharpener on hand. The cost is usually less than $5. I discuss skate sharpening more fully in the next chapter.

>  **TIP** Skate sharpening is a skilled job, which requires specialized equipment. Don't try to do it yourself. And except in an emergency, don't use those coin-operated sharpening machines. I think they do a terrible job.

STICKS

We have come a long way from the days when the Mi'kmaq of eastern Canada and the northeastern United States made sticks from trees, using the roots to form the blade. Today, a stick made of space-age composite materials can easily cost $100. Luckily, your child's first few sticks can be a lot cheaper than that. A standard, one-piece kid's stick, made of good, old-fashioned wood, is perfectly acceptable.

The key thing about a stick, though, is not the price or the material or the way it's made. It's the length. A stick that's too long or too short is going to hamper the player's game. It's as simple as that. Now, when you're in the store you'll be surrounded by hundreds of sticks that are all too long. Don't worry. The salespeople usually are kind enough to grab a hacksaw and cut the stick for you. Here's how to get the right length. Get your child to put on his or her skates. Then hold the stick vertically. With the blade toe on the ground, the tip of the shaft should be between the child's chin and nose. Once the stick is cut, your child should be able to move it back and forth in front of the body without getting the butt end hung up in the midsection and with the blade flat on the ice.

But there's more to sticks than getting the right length. You also have to consider size and curve. Sticks come in junior, intermediate and senior sizes. A junior stick has a small blade and a narrow shaft, suitable for tiny hands. Older kids use an intermediate stick, which is slightly bigger. Then, at about 12 or 13, it's time for a senior stick. Don't buy a senior stick, intending to cut it to the proper length for your 7-year-old. The shaft will be too thick and the blade too big.

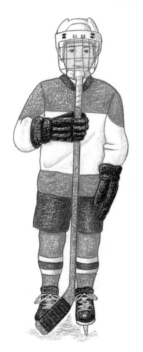

A Properly Sized Stick

With the skates on the child, the stick should end between the chin and the nose.

Then there's the curve of the blade. Stick blades are curved to allow a harder, more accurate shot on the forehand. The downside is that it's harder to control the puck when stick-handling, passing or taking a backhand shot. That's why I prefer—at least at first—straight blades for kids. Puck control is easier. Unfortunately, they can be very hard to find. Manufacturers, responding to the marketplace, make mostly curved sticks. So get the gentlest curve you can find. And, of course, make sure the curve matches the way your child shoots.

How do you know which way the child shoots? Easy. Give him or her a stick for a few minutes and watch. Pretty soon, you'll see which hand is preferred for the top and which for the shaft of the stick. Your child shoots left if the right hand is on the top of the stick and the left is on the shaft. And vice-versa for right.

There are all sorts of highly technical details about sticks that you may hear about. The lie of the stick, for example, refers to the angle between the blade and the shaft. An experienced player may prefer one lie over another, but your beginner probably has no preference (although he or she should have as much blade on the ice as possible). If your child goes on to play Midget or Junior, you will need to know about modern multi-piece sticks, where the shaft is aluminum or an almost unbreakable synthetic, and the replaceable blade is laminated wood. But until then, you need to worry about something much more down to earth. Taping the stick.

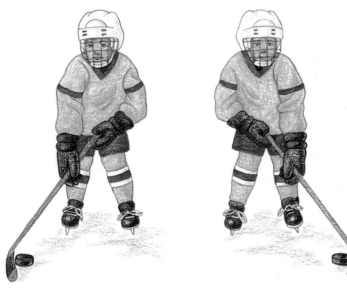

Does Your Child Shoot Right or Left?
The blade must curve the correct way.

The way a stick is taped can have a significant influence on your child's ability to control the puck. Most kids, especially beginners, have no idea how to go about it. You'll have to do it for your child, at least at first. I discuss the art of taping a stick at length in the next chapter. For now—just in case you're on the way to the sports shop—make sure you get white tape for the knob of the stick. The black stuff can absolutely ruin a hockey glove.

> **TIP** Sticks look alike. Print your child's name on the shaft with a marker.

A FEW TIPS ON THE REST OF THE EQUIPMENT

Now that we've covered buying helmets, skates and sticks, I'll give you some tips on buying and fitting the rest of the equipment. In the first few years in hockey, children don't need a whole lot of protection. Mostly, the gear is to protect against accidents—inadvertent collisions and the unavoidable tumbles onto the backside.

With that in mind, avoid bulky gear. I see some parents buying the top-line, pro model of every piece of equipment. This is fine for a player at the 14-year-old level, where body-checking is allowed and some of the kids stand six-foot-two and have already been shaving for two years. But for the first years, light, streamlined gear is best. It will protect your child, while at the same time allowing a full range of motion. Avoiding the pro models will also protect your pocketbook, since they tend to be expensive.

Again, make sure you bring your child with you when you're buying equipment. I learned that the hard way—by having to return equipment that didn't fit. And you can save yourself a lot of time by buying from a reputable sporting goods store. If you go to a discount store, you're likely to get a discount salesperson whose knowledge of hockey is minimal. That said, there's nothing wrong with trying to find used equipment, and there are excellent stores that specialize in used sporting goods. As well, some hockey associations have equipment exchange days at the beginning of the season.

The main thing to watch out for with used equipment is excessive wear. Examine the stitching and padding before you buy, looking for broken threads or torn and crushed padding. You are not really saving anything if you compromise protection. Many parents try to save money by buying oversized equipment, hoping to make it last a couple of seasons. This is *not* a good idea. Gear that's too big will make it hard for your child to play the game. And it won't protect as well as properly fitted equipment.

There are many different hockey equipment makers. Don't feel you have to buy the same brand for every piece of gear. But try to stick to the major manufacturers—CCM, Bauer, Hespeler, Easton, Jofa or Koho. You'll find that some brands of shin pads, say, will fit your child better than others, while yet another brand of gloves may do the trick. It all depends on your kid's body. That's why it's good to buy from a store that has a wide selection.

Next to the Skin: Underwear and Socks

Some parents let their kids wear street clothes under their hockey gear. Don't. The equipment has to fit snugly, and it won't with street clothes underneath. Sporting goods stores sell one-piece undergarments designed for hockey. Or you can use thin cotton pajamas. The underwear absorbs sweat and helps keep the equipment dry. It will also minimize odor build-up in the equipment.

Socks should be thin cotton. I think sweat socks are too thick; the skate and foot should be like a single unit. I also like to keep extra pairs in the hockey bag because you never know when holes will appear. Wash them after each use, of course. Some players feel more comfortable in bare feet. No problem as long as the skates are sized properly. Going barefoot certainly didn't slow down the great Bobby Orr.

The Jock and the Jill

The jock is a hard plastic cup, held in position by a cloth pouch, that protects the genitals. It's technically referred to as an athletic supporter and cup. (There are also various kinds of jock/garter combinations, about which more later.) These items are sized according to waist measurement; the jock should fit snugly but not so tightly as to be uncomfortable.

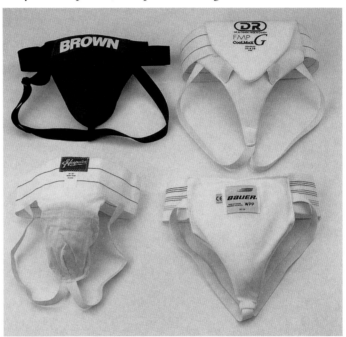

Jocks and Jills

The jocks are on the left and the jills on the right. The goalie versions are on top.

The protective cups come in different sizes. Make sure the one you buy fully covers your son's genitals. But remember. If the cup is too large, it will interfere with skating and will chafe the inside of the thighs.

The corresponding protective device for girls is called a jill. The jill-strap (or pelvic protector) is a padded, triangular piece of hard plastic and is sized according to waist measurement. Generally you'll only get a choice between a junior and a senior model. There are also special jills with more padding for goaltenders.

In the early years—before the shots get hard and the kids learn to raise the puck—your daughter may be more comfortable with a standard athletic supporter (minus the hard cup) and some foam padding. This would be the case if she's small and finds even a junior-sized jill to be too large. But it is important to have some sort of pelvic protection, because even at the earliest level of hockey, accidents can happen.

Shin Pads

Kids grow quickly, and you'll probably find your budding hockey player needs new shin pads at the beginning of every season. So you're looking at paying about $30 or $40 (or more) every autumn. On the plus side, the other players are growing out of shin pads every year, too. So you can usually find good used pads for much less than the price of new ones.

Shin pads should really be called shin-and-knee pads, because that's what they protect. Most also have soft padding that wraps around the calf. To get the right size, measure (in inches) the distance from the middle of your child's kneecap to just above the ankle bone. Pads are sized in inches, so it's just a matter of looking for a pair that matches the distance you just measured. Most pads will have the size in inches marked on them.

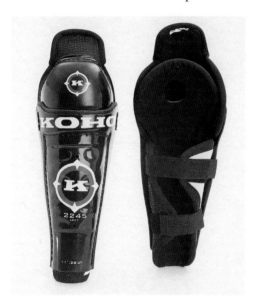

Shin Pads

A shin pad protects the front and side of the lower leg.

Kids have small knees and calves, so make sure the pad is not too broad or it can interfere with the skater's stride. However, the padding should extend around the side of the knee for better protection. You are looking for a snug anatomic fit to the shin and calf. Also, look for brands with a flexible joint between the knee and shin.

Keep in mind that beginners don't need expensive bulky pads because their teammates and opponents still can't shoot very hard. However, a too-short pad puts your child in danger from stray pucks or sticks hitting the area near the ankle. If the pad is too long, on the other hand, your child won't be able to bend the ankle properly—and that will interfere with his or her skating.

I like shin pads with some thick felt extending from the bottom to protect the front of the ankle from the skate laces, which can dig in after they're tightened. Unfortunately, most manufacturers today just put a little bit of soft foam at the end of the pad. Some pads have doughnut-shaped padding in the knee, with a central cut-out that cups the kneecap. These fit—and protect—better than others. Some shin pads also come with an air bladder system that helps absorb impacts. These aren't much more expensive than regular pads but, again, I think they're not necessary at this age.

Most shin pads today also have straps attached to make sure the pad is held snugly in place. You can also buy straps if the pads you've bought don't have them. And many players like to tape their pads in place over the hockey socks. (Hockey shops sell a clear plastic tape. Use this instead of the cloth tape, which is more expensive and can cause holes in the socks.)

The Garter Belt and Hockey Socks

The garter belt is so named because … well … it is a garter belt. Its job is to hold up the hockey socks. Hockey garter belts are fitted according to waist size, and they come with four adjustable clips that attach to the socks. Most kids will need help attaching them, because they're a bit tricky. You can get a garter belt already attached to the jockstrap, which eliminates having two things around the waist.

A recently introduced product combines the jockstrap with the garter in a one-piece arrangement. The hockey socks stick to Velcro strips on the outside of a pair of shorts that contain the protective cup. There is also a jill version.

> **TIP** Don't tape around the top of the socks to hold them up, something I see done all the time. The tape will interfere with blood flow and muscle contraction in the thigh.

The hockey socks—thick, woven affairs—are there to hold the shin pads in place. If they're correctly sized, they should reach to the upper third of the thigh. If the socks are too long, you can cut them down and sew another seam along the top. And while we're talking about sewing, repair holes as soon as they appear—and they will appear—or you'll find yourself buying a new

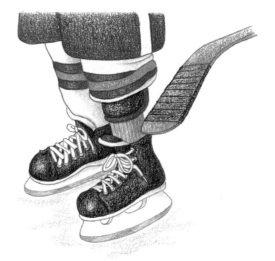

Too-short Shin Pad
A shin pad that's too short will leave the ankles exposed to injury.

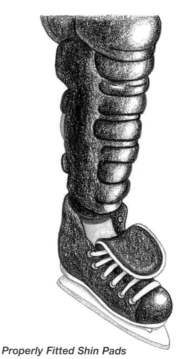

Properly Fitted Shin Pads
A properly fitted shin pad protects the lower shin without interfering with ankle movement.

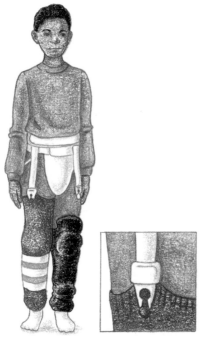

Garter Belts

Kids will need help attaching their garter belts to the socks. The inset shows how the clip attaches to the sock.

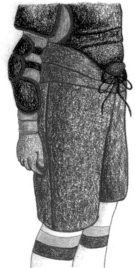

Hockey Pants

The upper part of the pants should meet the shoulder pads and the lower part should meet the kneecap.

pair pretty quickly. Many hockey associations will supply socks at the start of the year, colored to match the team jerseys.

Hockey Pants

Hockey pants will usually last a child two seasons. Used pants will probably be fine; they have a long lifespan. But do inspect used pants carefully to make sure all the stitching and padding are intact. Used ones will, as usual, be cheaper than new ones.

Hockey pants are sized by waist measurement—usually between 4 and 6 inches larger than your child's actual waist. The key test is this: The player should be able to squat with the hockey pants on. If he or she can't, the pants are too small. The pants protect the thigh, the pelvic and hip bones, the kidneys and the lower ribs. Obviously, to do that, they have to cover those areas. So they should come down to mid-kneecap and up to the bottom third of the chest.

Look for pants with good padding over the tailbone. Players who are learning the game will fall a lot, usually on their behinds. Different brands of pants will fit differently, so try several pairs to see which one fits your child best. Most pants today come with a belt that tightens around the waist, but they can also be held up the old way with suspenders if your child prefers.

Pants will absorb a lot of moisture during a game or practice, because, as I said, most new players fall a lot. So it's important that the pants be hung up to dry after every use. This will prolong their lifespan, making it easier to hand them on to a younger sibling or to resell them at a garage sale.

Shoulder Pads

Particularly in the first couple of years, go for lightweight, streamlined shoulder pads, with enough room for your child to move his or her shoulders freely. But the pads should fit snugly, allowing easy movement of the upper body for skating, shooting and puck control. Most shoulder pads will last your child two seasons. Used shoulder pads are relatively easy to find, because they tend to last; they're also cheaper, of course.

The shoulder pads protect the chest, shoulders, upper back and upper arms. In front, the shoulder pads should cover the chest down to just below the nipples, where they should meet the pants. The arm padding should meet or overlap the top of the elbow pad. The plastic shoulder cap should rest over the point of the shoulder.

The Hespeler Hockey Co. has come up with something called a cardiac guard. This attaches to the shoulder pad to provide extra protection to the heart. Some Hespeler shoulder pads come with the cardiac guard attached. In principle, this sounds good. But, as a doctor, I haven't seen any definitive research to verify its effectiveness. Chest injuries are rare in hockey, especially in children's hockey, and it's unlikely anybody will have a shot hard enough and high enough to worry about. Let's remember that chest injuries from a projectile are far more likely in baseball. But except for the catcher, no ball players wear cardiac guards.

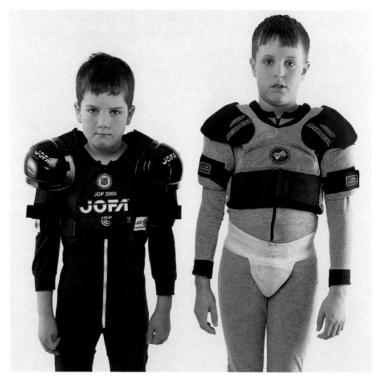

Shoulder Pads

Especially in the first years of hockey, avoid linebacker-style shoulder pads like those on the left. Good, lighter pads (like those on the right) are safe and allow for easier movement.

In the past few years, shoulder pads have undergone a drastic change. Many of today's pads are far too bulky, with too much padding. I have seen some kids playing hockey who look more like linebackers than defense players. The fact is that most kids don't need the heavy-duty, linebacker-style pads until they reach the age where body-checking is allowed. And I'm not sure they need them then. With huge shoulder pads, players start thinking they're invincible and start doing foolish things on the ice. The results, I think, are injuries that can be avoided.

Elbow Pads

Elbow pads will usually last a young player two and sometimes even three seasons. Buy good ones. Kids fall on their elbows a lot more than they do on their shoulders.

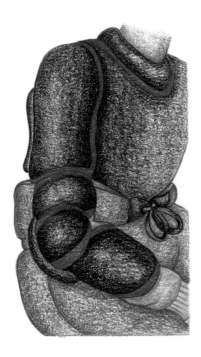

Sizing Elbow Pads

The elbow pad should protect from the middle of the upper arm to the middle of the forearm.

Used pads are, of course, cheaper than new. Make sure the padding is not worn or cracked.

Elbow pads should be long enough to protect from about the middle of the upper arm to the middle of the forearm, while fitting snugly around the elbow itself. They shouldn't be so tight that your child has trouble flexing or extending the elbow. I prefer pads that attach with Velcro straps (as long as the Velcro is in good shape) because they make it easier to get a snug fit. Whether the pads are new or used, be aware that the Velcro on the straps tends to wear with time. Make sure it will stay closed, because you don't want the pad shifting during a game.

Also make sure the pads have a doughnut-shaped cup for the point of the elbow. I like elbow pads with a slash guard—an extension that covers the forearm and fits inside the top of the hockey glove. You *can* buy separate slash guards, but why? They're another piece of equipment to get lost. The goal here is to make sure the forearm is protected. If the elbow pad and glove are sized correctly, separate slash guards shouldn't be needed. (That said, I suggest you read the next section on gloves before going out to buy elbow pads.)

The outer shell of the pads can be made of plastic or leather, but for kids I prefer leather. It just fits better. Plastic shells are now illegal in the NHL because they do contribute to injuries (I hope the manufacturers will stop making them). If you want to buy top-line equipment, I suggest spending the money on elbow pads rather than shoulder pads. It's much more likely your child will fall on the elbow than the shoulder.

Hockey Gloves

Gloves are my favorite piece of equipment. They are the key to proper puck-handling—if your child has thick, heavy gloves and can't feel the stick through the palms, there's no way he or she will be able to stick-handle, pass or shoot. Sadly, I see many kids with just that problem. Walter Gretzky, father of the famous Wayne, always believed in buying light equipment for his children. Indeed, to the end of his NHL career, Wayne Gretzky preferred light equipment that let him use his awesome skills (although he did use gloves with long cuffs to protect against slashes to the forearm and wrist).

Today's gloves are, for the most part, pretty light, and there's no compromise with protection. So you can safely look for light gloves with pliable palms. Again, gloves

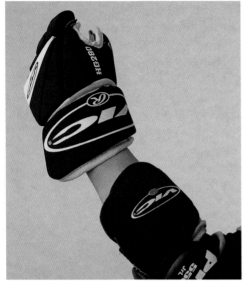 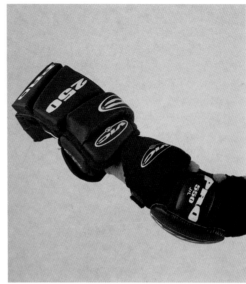

Hockey Gloves

The glove on the left is a great way to end your kid's season, while the glove on the right affords proper forearm protection.

last, so a used pair is a definite possibility. If you're looking for used gloves, make sure the palms and fingers are intact.

The gloves should be snug but not tight. They are sized in inches. An average 7-year-old, for instance, will fit into a 10- or 11-inch glove. But that's only an average, so make sure the child is with you when you buy gloves. (The smallest glove size I have ever seen, by the way, is 8-inch.) The top of the glove should reach the middle of the forearm, and there should be no gap between the end of the glove and the beginning of the elbow pad. Some gloves sold today are in the short-cuff style. As a doctor and a coach, I think these gloves leave too much of the forearm and wrist exposed and should be avoided. Gloves with a regular cuff length have quite enough flexibility and still offer protection. But if your child insists on short-cuffed gloves, make sure he or she wears slash guards to protect the exposed area. These are like elasticized sweatbands for the wrist and can be purchased at sporting goods stores.

To break in the gloves, let your child wear them playing road hockey (or even wear them around the house for a few days). A new pair should be used in practice first, not in actual games.

TIP   Gloves need to be air dried after use to prolong their life and prevent the palms from cracking.

Neck Guards

While neck guards are not required equipment in the United States, they are mandatory in Canada. The protection offered by neck guards is well worth the expense, so if you're north of the border pick one up. They protect the windpipe and the major blood vessels in the neck from accidental cuts or blows. Despite what

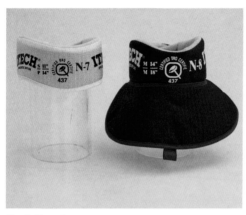

Neck Guards

The neck guard (which is mandatory in Canada) protects the windpipe and neck arteries, but *not* the spine. The one on the right has a bib and is usually worn by goalies.

anyone might tell you, a neck guard does *not* protect the spine. There are two types—a simple cushion affair that wraps around the neck, and a larger version that has a short, stiff bib down the front. Make sure you get a neck guard that is certified by the Bureau de Normalisation du Quebec (the B.N.Q. label should be on the guard). The B.N.Q. is the only agency that has set standards for neck guards; others aren't approved by most hockey associations.

Neck guards are sized according to the neck size, and they come in extra small, small, medium, large and extra large. They must fit snugly, covering the entire front of the neck. Because they have Velcro closures, they can be adjusted to fit. They do last well, but they should be replaced if the Velcro becomes worn; you don't want them shifting during play.

For information on the throat guards worn by goalies, turn to Chapter 6.

Hockey Bags

Finally, you're going to need to tote all this equipment around. Invest in a good quality hockey bag. It will last for years.

Look for a bag with skate pockets on the side and a separate pouch for the various small bits, such as a skate towel, underwear, tape (white, black and clear), skate hone, skate guards, screwdriver, extra screws for the helmet, water bottle, stick wax, and asthma medicine (if necessary). A puck and a tennis ball aren't a bad idea either—you never know when or where an impromptu game of shinny might break out.

Keep a small piece of carpet at the bottom of the bag so your child has a dry area to stand on while changing. All those snow-covered skate blades can make a mess of a dressing room floor.

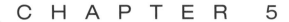

CHAPTER 5

The Equipment
Preparation and Maintenance

TAKING CARE OF THE EQUIPMENT

Proper care will prolong the life of your child's hockey equipment. And that means you can sell it or trade it next year. Or hand it on to the next child in line.

Equipment should be aired out at room temperature after every game and practice. Many hardware and sporting goods stores sell special airing racks that you can set up in the corner of the basement. Hockey pants in particular (along with the socks and jersey) will absorb a lot of moisture during a game or practice, because most new players fall a lot. So it's important to hang the pants up to dry after every use.

Remember, gloves need to be air dried after use to prolong their life and prevent the palms from cracking. By the way, unless it's a jersey, socks or underwear, don't put any equipment in the clothes dryer—the high temperatures can break down the equipment, especially gloves.

Whatever you do, don't make the mistake of leaving the gear in the car all season. Mold and bacteria will proliferate and begin to break down the equipment. And your child will be sitting alone on the dressing room bench. Most equipment can be washed by hand. Gently scrub it with some mild soap and water and let it air dry. The dryer is a bad idea.

If—like me—you have more time on your hands than is good for you, you can even build your own change room. I remodeled a room off our basement, so that we each have our own stall, with hooks for equipment. There's also room for our hockey collectibles and awards. This, I freely admit, is excessive.

TAPING THE STICK

I have always enjoyed taping a hockey stick. I go slowly and I take a lot of pride in doing it properly. Since it will be you the parent doing it for the next year or two at least, you might as well start out the right way. Two points first off. Make sure you buy hockey tape—a specialized product made of cloth—rather than shiny black electrical tape. (I see many new hockey parents making this mistake.) And never use black tape to make the grip on the upper shaft of the stick. It can ruin a hockey glove.

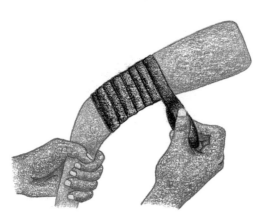

Taping the Blade
Start at the heel and work toward the toe.

Hockey tape comes in a range of colors, although black and white are the most common and all you'll ever need. Remember that the tape will wear fairly quickly, especially on the bottom. Inspect it regularly and redo as needed.

The idea behind taping is to improve the contact between the stick and the puck, and also to help protect the blade. Begin by running a strip of tape along the bottom of the blade. Then, starting at the heel of the blade, wrap the tape around, with each turn overlapping the previous one by about half the width of the tape. Keep the tape as smooth as possible. Once you are finished, press the tape down with your hand or a puck. Some players like to rub wax on the blade to repel snow and water and prolong the life of the tape.

Next you need to put a knob and a grip on the end of the shaft. The knob is like the flared ridge on the end of a baseball bat; it prevents the stick from sliding out of the player's hands. The knob is *not* meant to be held in the hand; make sure your child holds the stick below the knob on the grip that you've taped. You make the knob by winding tape around the end of the shaft. And winding tape around the shaft. And winding tape around ... You get the idea. You make the grip by twisting the tape so it forms a string; while twisting, wind it around the stick in a spiral pattern. Then wrap a single layer of tape over that. What does the grip do? Well, it improves the player's grip. Some players—like me—prefer not to have a knob and just hold the stick at the end on the grip.

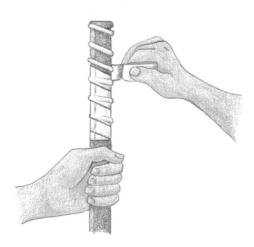

Taping the Knob and Grip
Don't make the knob too big for small hands. Make the grip long enough for the entire gloved hand, about five inches.

I have three pieces of advice. Make the knob relatively small at first, because your child's hands are small. (It should be large enough, however, that if the stick is dropped your child can pick it up off the ice fairly easily with gloved hands.) Make sure the grip extends at least a few inches down the shaft so that there's enough room for the whole glove. And use white tape if you want to keep the glove's palm in good shape.

Lastly, I'll tell you once more. Sticks look alike. Take a marker and put your child's name somewhere on the shaft.

SHARPENING THE SKATES

Skates need to be sharpened regularly. The first time to do it is as soon as you buy them—new or used. Some sporting goods shops and most hockey shops and arenas have skate-sharpening equipment and personnel. The cost is nominal. Skate sharpening requires a fair amount of skill, so I wouldn't suggest doing it yourself. Some rinks have coin-operated sharpeners; they're not worth the trouble in my view. Take the skates to a pro.

Sharpening the skates involves grinding a groove down the length of the blade, creating an inside and an outside edge; if they start to get uneven or pick up dings and dents, get them resharpened. Get used to the way sharp skates feel. The edges should be even and without nicks or gouges as you gently rub a finger *across* the edges (not along them, unless you like having cut fingers). There'll be a little bit of drag against your skin. Once that feeling is gone, the skates need another sharpening. You'll sometimes hear coaches or parents talk about "losing an edge," which means the skate has been dulled. One sign of a lost edge is that the player is slipping and falling on turns or when trying to push off.

In my experience, most parents tend to let their child's skates get dull. My guess is kids can usually skate between six and eight hours before they need their skates sharpened. Still, that's only a rough guideline. Kids

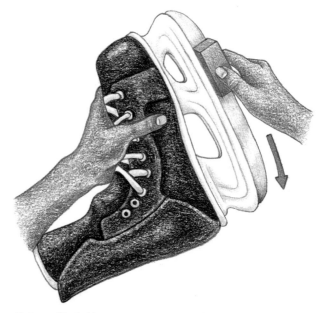

Using a Skate Hone
A full-scale sharpening may not be needed every time. A skate hone can take off a little nick or gouge.

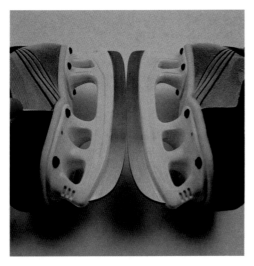

The Rocker
The skate blades are rockered (or curved); if they weren't you wouldn't be able to turn. Only a portion of the blade is in contact with the ice at any time.

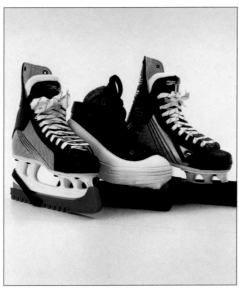

Skate Guards
Skate guards protect the skates—and also the other equipment in the hockey bag.

step on all sorts of things that dull the blades. It's better to sharpen skates before they absolutely need it.

If there's just a little nick in recently sharpened skates, you don't need the full treatment. Get a hone (a hockey whetstone, available at the pro shop) and rub it along the nicked side of the blade. Often you can remove the gouge without a full-scale sharpening. If you're not comfortable doing this, ask the coach or a knowledgable parent to show you for the first time.

From time to time, you'll hear a lot of jargon about skate sharpening. For instance, you'll hear the term "rockered." All this means is that the blades are not flat, but curved like the runner of a rocking chair. Hold the blades up together and you'll see what I mean. The amount of the curve or rocker is also known as the skate's profile or radius. You'll also hear the term "radius hollow," which refers to the groove created by the sharpening machine. Hold the sharpened skate up and look along the blade—you'll easily see the groove. The deeper the groove, the sharper the edges. At the top levels of hockey, different rockers and radius grooves are important; players have distinct preferences, depending on how they play the game. But in the first few years of hockey, unless your child is playing a lot of goal, it's unlikely to matter much (I discuss goalies' skates more in Chapter 6).

Skates will dull faster if your child is skating on natural outdoor ice. They'll also dull more quickly if they're not kept covered by skate guards off the ice. And they'll lose their edge if they rust, so keep a small towel in the hockey bag to wipe the blades off after play.

BE PREPARED FOR ANYTHING

Here's a review of some of the tips I gave along the way, plus a few new ones.

- If you keep a little square of carpet in the hockey bag, your child can stand on it while changing. Dressing room floors can get very messy because of the ice left on skates and sticks after a game. Keep in mind that the floor can be wet *before* a game if you're in a dressing room that has just been used by another team.

- Rust build-up on skate blades can be prevented by wiping them after each use. Keep a small towel in the hockey bag for this purpose. This also helps keep moisture and mildew out of the rest of the equipment in the bag. Remember to take the towel out at home so that it can dry.

- Unless they're wearing rubber boots, children's socks may get wet when it's snowing or raining outside. It's better not to wear wet socks (or ones with holes) inside skates, especially if the rink happens to be a very cold one. So keep an extra pair in the bag.

- Always keep an extra roll of white hockey tape in the bag, and black too if you're also using it on the blade. Remember to use only white tape on the shaft and for the knob.

- Keep an extra shin-pad strap or two in the hockey bag if your child's pads require them. Also, keep some of the clear plastic tape in the bag if your child likes to tape the socks on over the shin pads. Don't use regular hockey tape over the socks—the tape is more expensive and can tear the fabric.

- Repair holes in hockey socks as soon as they appear, or you'll be buying new ones very soon.

- Laces snap and wear out. Keep an extra set in the bag.

- Keep a screwdriver handy since the facemask will occasionally loosen from the helmet. Having a few extra screws in the bag isn't a bad idea either.

Pregame Equipment Checklist

(The goalie checklist appears at the end of the next chapter.)

Age: _____

Weight: _____

Height: _____

____ Underwear	____ Shoulder pads
____ Thin cotton socks	____ Neck guard
____ Jock/Jill	____ Helmet
____ Garter belt	____ Facemask
____ Shin pads	____ Visor cleaner (for clear plastic shield masks)
____ Hockey socks	____ Mouth guard (mandatory in U.S.A. from Peewee up)
____ Hockey pants	____ Gloves
____ Skates	____ Stick
____ Skate guards	____ Hockey bag
____ Elbow pads	

In addition to the main equipment items listed above, here are some suggestions for other items to keep in the hockey bag. Being prepared can make your life a lot simpler.

Extras

Extra underwear, extra socks, tape (black, white and clear), skate hone, skate towel, laces, screwdriver, extra screws for the helmet, water bottle, stick wax, and asthma medicine if it's needed. You can keep a puck and a tennis or hockey ball in the bag, too.

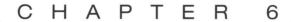

My Kid Wants to Play Goal

As a hockey player, coach and all-around fan, I find everything about the game fascinating, but when it came to goaltending I was in the same boat as you. I too am a first-time hockey parent ... of a goalie.

When Spencer, my middle son, announced his desire to be a goalie, I was thunderstruck. I knew a lot about kids and a lot about the other hockey positions, but not very much about the masked player between the pipes.

Luckily, I do know a few things about hockey. One of the most important things I've learned over the years is this: If you don't know, ask someone who does. I turned to Pat Maloney, who owns Sports Unlimited, a hockey store in Brampton, Ontario, near where I practice medicine. Pat is an expert on goaltending equipment, which is completely different from the gear worn by the other players. He also has a son who plays goal, so he was able to alert me to some of what lies ahead for Spencer and for me.

In the first few years of hockey, it's unlikely your son or daughter will play goal all the time. Good coaches like to spread the goaltending duties around, and that's as it should be. I see some coaches pick the worst skater on the team and stick him or her in net. This is not a good idea. How can a child learn to skate while standing in the net? The first aim for the kids should be to learn to skate and handle the puck. Once a player commits to playing goal, he or she will work on skills that only goaltenders rely on. Don't rush into it. There will be time enough to specialize later on.

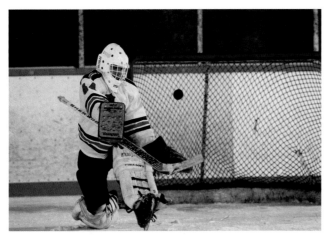

NHL Goalie in Action

Maybe it's the specialized equipment that makes the position of goaltender attractive to some kids.

But suppose your child has the fixed notion of being a goaltender. Maybe the idea springs from playing road hockey. Or maybe he or she just likes the equipment—the huge pads, the streamlined mask, the big flat stick. My advice then is to do what I'm doing—go with it.

But try to make sure your child gets some time out of the net, so he or she can develop skating, shooting and puck-handling skills. One year, I helped coach a Tyke team that had two kids who wanted to play goal. We used to alternate them, and the one not in net for that game would take a regular shift as a skater. Spencer's Tyke coach did the same thing, and I believe that all coaches should do this with very young players.

Two other points may worry you: the cost of goalie equipment, and the danger of the position. Yes, the equipment can be very expensive, but there are ways to make it affordable. The first thing to remember is that you probably won't have to buy everything, especially if your child is playing at the earlier levels of hockey. The house league will, in all likelihood, supply some equipment. Most leagues, for example, supply the big pads, the stick and some other equipment for games. As to the second point, no, the position is not more dangerous than others, especially with today's equipment. Also, in these early years the skaters aren't very fast and the shots are soft.

THE EQUIPMENT

If your child is playing goal, someone will have to help him or her get dressed. It might as well be you, so here's a quick guide to the gear, starting from the skin out.

As with skaters, the goalie should not wear street clothes under the pads. Instead, use a one-piece hockey undergarment or even a pair of cotton pajamas.

Next to go on is the jock or jill. Goalies wear extra-protective jocks (or jills) with a lot of extra padding, but in the first years, the regular equipment will do. After all, the shots are not likely to be very hard. (There's a picture of jocks and jills for skaters and goalies in Chapter 4.)

Then come the socks. One difference with goalies is that the hockey socks go on before those bulky goal pads. Hold the socks up with a garter belt—the same as the skaters use.

Next to go on are the pants. There are special hockey pants for goalies with—you guessed it—more padding. But for the early years, use regular hockey pants; the goalie can maneuver more easily. If your child still wants to be a goalie in a few years (when the shots start getting harder), goalie pants are a must.

Now come the skates. There are specialized goalie skates, but not for young kids. When your child is about 9, he or she might be ready for goal skates. It depends on foot size. The smallest goalie skates start at Junior size 2 or 3. Goalie skates have special blades, as well as very stiff boots—sometimes reinforced with Kevlar—for extra protection. That said, your child's regular skates will be fine, at least for the early years.

I should add that the blades of goal skates are ground differently than regular skates. In Chapter 5 on equipment, I mentioned that regular skate blades are curved, or rockered. Goal skate blades are flatter and wider, which makes it easier for the goalie to slide from side to side in the crease. If your child is going to play in net exclusively, you might have the skate rocker flattened. (The skate sharpener can do it.) If the child is going to play both goal and some other position, you could even pick up a spare pair of skates (new or used). Keep one pair ground for the goal and the other for forward or defense.

The goalie—like other players—must wear a wraparound neck protector. Goalie neck guards extend like a bib over the collarbone and upper part of the breastbone for added protection. This is different from the throat shield, which I'll talk about in a moment, along with the helmets.

The chest and arm pads can go on next (or you can wait until you've strapped on the goalie pads). These complicated pieces of padding (usually one-piece these days) should cover the entire chest and belly (down to the top of the jock or jill), the upper back, the collarbone, the upper arms and part of the forearms.

Make sure the pads come down far enough on the arm so there's no gap between them and the blocker and catching glove. The idea here is to make sure the arms, chest and spine

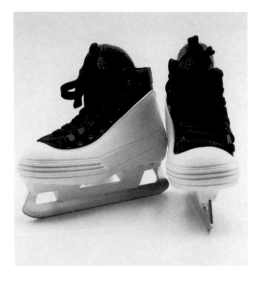

Goal Skates

Goal skates have flat blades and extra-heavy protective boots, but they're not made in small sizes.

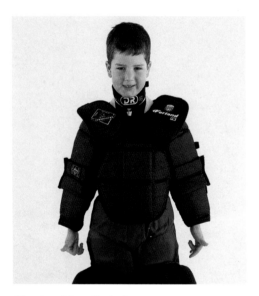

Chest and Arm Protector

The chest and arm protector comes as a one-piece unit. It must cover all of the chest, abdomen and arms since these are potential injury areas from incoming shots.

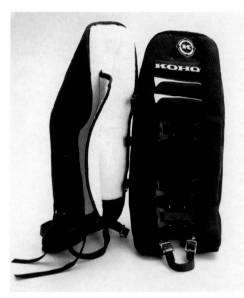

Goalie Pads

The heavy pads protect the goalie from incoming shots. It may take your child a while to learn to maneuver in this heavy equipment.

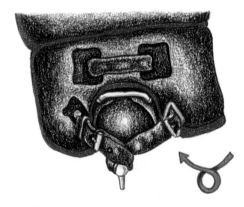

The Toe Buckle

The toe strap should criss-cross or wrap around the front of the skate holder. Buckle it up as tightly as possible.

are all padded in any place the puck might possibly hit—and that's just about anywhere.

Goalie leg pads, which are sized in inches, come in all sizes, shapes, materials and colors, but if you're using the league's pads, you'll pretty much have to take what you get. That said, make sure they cover the entire lower leg, from the top of the skate to about four inches above the knee. The pants slip in behind the top of the pad, providing protection all the way up.

There is a left and right to goalie pads. Each pad has a vertical roll of padding down one edge; this is the outside.

Put the pads on the floor, have the goalie kneel down on them and then have him or her lie face forward on the floor, while you attach the calf straps. Different makes of pads have different strap arrangements, but the rule of thumb is this: The bottom straps should be tight, to minimize slippage, while the top ones should be looser so the goalie isn't too restricted in his or her movements.

There will also be a buckle at the bottom of each pad to attach it to the skate. Many parents simply loop the leather strap through the front hole of the blade holder. This is incorrect and will leave the pads too loose and difficult to maneuver in. The strap is usually attached on the outside of the toe opening of the pad. Take the strap and cross it over the front of the blade holder so it enters the front hole of the blade holder from the opposite side (the inside). Then pull it through; when you buckle it on to the other side of the toe opening, the strap will have made a criss-cross at the front of the skate and be wrapped around underneath it. It should be buckled as tightly as possible. If you're unsure how to do it, get another parent or the coach to show you the first time.

Slip the jersey on over the padding. You may need an oversize one to cover the chest protector; your association should have one, perhaps from the next age group up.

Next comes the helmet and mask. If you've ever watched the NHL, you'll have noticed the streamlined masks, decorated with logos or snarling predators, worn by the goalies. If your child decides to play goal exclusively, it's only a matter of time until you'll be asked for one of these.

In the meantime, don't allow him or her to paint the goalie mask. This can void manufacturer warranties.

Up until about 40 years ago, of course, no goalie would have dreamed of wearing a mask. Now, no goalie would dream of not wearing one. And parents of young goalies would scream if anyone suggested such a thing. (I wonder what parents of goalies thought back then.)

The streamlined, form-fitting mask offers the most protection. It distributes impact well, fits snugly so that it doesn't shift, and deflects most pucks away from the face. But it's also expensive and heavy; for young children, you don't need to spend the money.

In fact, most young kids just need a regular helmet and wire facemask, the same gear they'd use if they were playing forward, at least until the age of 13 or 14. That said, there are wire facemasks that are specially designed for goalies. If you buy one, buy it new. As I say in Chapter 4, I don't like used helmets or facemasks, because you don't know their history. Also, make sure you get an approved helmet and facemask. In the United States look for the HECC seal, and in Canada look for the CSA approval sticker.

Goalies are more susceptible to injuries around the neck from pucks, skates and sticks, so a throat shield is important (regular players don't require one). A throat guard is a hinged shield made of clear plastic that hangs in front of the neck. They're tricky to attach, so you might want to get the store personnel to show you how it's done. And if the child wears the same helmet while playing another position, don't forget to take it off. By the way, even with a throat shield, the goalie must wear a neck guard, too.

Before every game and practice, inspect the mask and helmet to make sure all the screws and fasteners are tight.

That's it for the equipment, except for the gloves and stick.

Unlike the forward and defense players, goalies wear two very different gloves. One has a flat, hard piece of plastic attached to the back of the glove, while the other features a big basket, like a huge first baseman's mitt.

The first one is the blocker. It's worn on the stick hand and it's used—as the name suggests—to block shots or

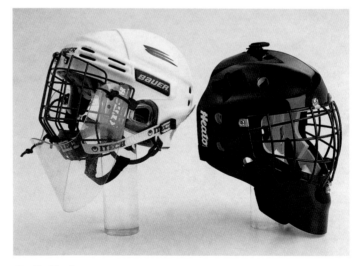

Goalie Masks
The one on the left is a regular player's helmet and wire mask with the throat shield attached. Throat shields are important but they're tricky to attach; ask sports store personnel to show you how it's done. The one on the right is a specialized mask for goalies.

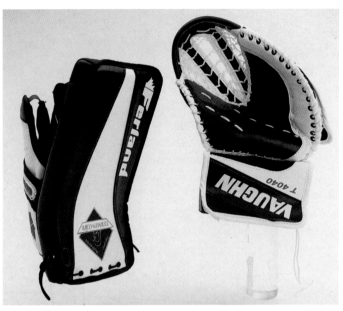

Goalie Gloves

The blocker (left) is used to deflect shots away; the catcher (right) is used to snag airborne pucks or smother loose pucks and rebounds.

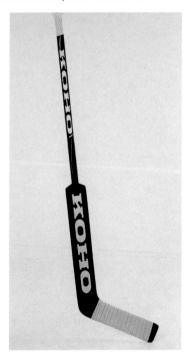

The Goalie Stick

The wide blade of the stick continues up the shaft (where it is called the paddle). The shoulder is the top part of the paddle where it meets the narrow shaft. Most goalies use white tape for the knob and on the blade.

knock them away. Your league will probably have various blockers available. Make sure the one your child picks doesn't have too much room in the fingers. If it does, he or she will have trouble controlling the stick. Also make sure there is enough space for the arm pads to fit comfortably under the top end of the blocker.

The other glove is simply called the trapper or the catcher. It is used—as its appearance suggests—to catch flying pucks and smother loose pucks on the ice. In fact, I remember as a kid using my ball glove when I played goal in road hockey games.

Today's blockers and trappers are technological marvels. Made of synthetic leather and nylon, they have features to deaden rebounds, special thumb pieces to direct a puck into the pocket, and hinge devices to allow greater wrist mobility. Your child, though, will probably be using the league's gloves and will have to make do without state-of-the-art puck-stopping technology. The most important thing, then, is fit and feel. Gloves that are too big will be hard to handle; a trapper or blocker that is too small won't stop as many pucks (and isn't as safe).

The last piece of specialized goal equipment is the stick. Unlike players' sticks, goalie sticks cannot be bought and cut to size. They're carefully balanced by the maker, which means you need to have your child with you when selecting one. Whether you are supplied one by your association (a normal practice because they're expensive) or you're buying one, here's what you need to know. The goalie stick has a wider blade, and this wide portion of the stick continues about one-third of the way up the shaft. The wide portion on the shaft is referred to as the paddle. The length of the paddle will vary, depending on the manufacturer and the size of the stick. Where the paddle ends and the regular shaft begins is called the shoulder. The paddle length is important because it determines where on the shaft your child will hold the stick. Too often parents, thinking that a larger stick will stop more pucks, will buy a stick that's too big and limits their child's ability to maneuver. When selecting one for your child, do it with the skates, pads, catcher and blocker on. This way, with your child in the goalie stance (it's also called the crouch), you can see if the stick and paddle are the right size. In the stance, the stick blade is flat on the ice, the blocker and trapper hands are each held at about waist level, the knees are bent and the goalie is slightly flexed forward at the waist. If the blocker hand can't get to the right level because the paddle comes too high on the shaft, then the stick is too big. On the other hand, if the paddle is too short the blocker will come too low on the shaft and disrupt your child's balance. As for overall length, the end of the shaft should be at about shoulder height when your child is in the stance.

As for the quality, like most other things, you get what you pay for. A cheap stick will wear out quickly because it is almost constantly being banged on the ice. Buy a good one; it will also be lighter and possibly reinforced with Kevlar or graphite.

Tape the stick with white tape using the same technique I describe for players' sticks (see Chapter 5), except for the knob. Avoid black tape on the blade since it makes it harder for referees and goal judges to see the black puck against the stick. It's also easier for the goalie to see the puck against the blade in the heat of action. In some leagues (like the NHL),

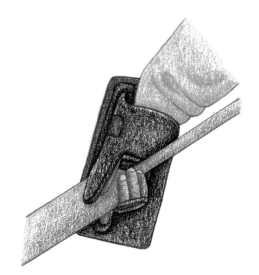

Holding the Stick

The goalie holds the stick at the shoulder, just above the paddle. The thumb should be placed flat on the upper part of the paddle, and the index finger should press against the other side of the paddle. This prevents the stick from rotating when stopping pucks.

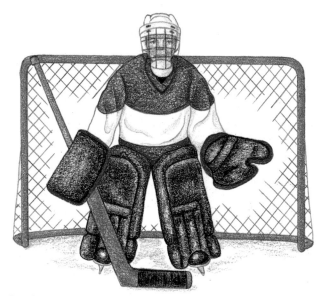

The Goalie Stance

When the stick blade is flat on the ice, the blocker and trapper hands should be at the same level, and the end of the stick should be at shoulder height. Note that the hand sits at the top of the paddle (near the stick's "shoulder").

it's a rule that the knob of the goal stick must be taped in white (a goal judge could mistake a black knob for a puck inside the net). Make the knob oversized: It prevents the stick from flying out of the goalie's hand during a poke-check. Also, a large knob makes it easier to pick the stick up if it's dropped because it doesn't lie flat on the ice.

If your child likes to play goal, you may find that—like me—you have spawned a budding Curtis Joseph or Ken Dryden. Then you'll have to decide how much you want to invest in his or her hockey career. Because—make no mistake—goalie equipment is expensive.

That said, you can keep the cost down by buying used gear. As with used gear for regular players, check to make sure the equipment isn't damaged, the padding worn or the stitching broken. You can expect to pay about half the retail price. The goalie pads, however, may be a bit more. And don't compromise on the mask and helmet—buy new.

THE PSYCHOLOGY

Playing goal is a tough job, both physically and mentally. I want to talk for just a moment about the mental aspect of the position.

Goaltending is the most difficult position to play in hockey. As I mentioned earlier, good coaches will have all the kids try the position at least once—then players will appreciate how difficult it really is. Goalies occasionally become the focus of criticism from other players. This must not be tolerated. The team as a whole is responsible for a win or a loss—never just the goalie. What's a good response to a player complaining about all the shots the goalie let in? Ask why the attacking players were allowed to get so close to the net on all those occasions. It's tough for goalies. They'll never score the goal that ties or wins the game, but they'll let in the shot that loses it. The mistakes of most players (a missed pass, for example) have few direct consequences, but the goalie's mistakes appear on the score sheet. Even if the goalie has played a great game, he or she may be in tears after a loss. Take the time to remind your child that the whole game isn't on the goalie's shoulders. Beyond playing the best that he or she can, no one can ask for more.

If your child wants to play goal and you're worried not only about the mental burden but also about the expense, consider having your child attend a summer goalie camp for a week or so. That way, at least you'll be more certain about what he or she really wants before you spend all that money on equipment. Your local hockey association can probably be persuaded to let your child borrow some pads for the camp.

FITNESS FOR GOALIES

Goalies need to be more flexible than the other players. There are three stretches I like for goalies: the butterfly groin stretch or sitting groin stretch, the quadriceps stretch (while lying on the side) and the sitting hamstring stretch. (You'll find pictures of these stretches in Chapter 7.)

Goalies also have to develop muscle strength to shift those huge pads around quickly. If you have your own pads, have your child wear them around the house once in a while, especially when starting out. Or grab a hockey ball and take some practice shots on him or her in the basement or on the driveway.

If your child is serious about playing goal, he or she may have to work on foot speed and quickness. Other sports—such as soccer, tennis and racquetball—may be useful for this. The racket sports in particular are good for developing hand-eye coordination. Learning how to juggle, odd as it may seem, is another excellent way to develop goalie reflexes.

There are a few injuries that are more common in goalies than in the other players. (See Chapter 7 for a discussion of injury prevention.) The one you hear a lot about is the groin pull. Usually what happens is the goalie does the splits trying to stop a puck, and one of the muscles in the groin tears slightly. The only real treatment is rest and physiotherapy; if your child does pull a groin muscle, make sure it's completely healed before letting him or her back in the net. Working on the splits greatly increases flexibility and reduces the risk of this injury. However, don't give your child the impression that he or she will be able to do the splits in a day or two. It can take months to develop flexibility in that area—so don't rush it.

The goalie is very often down on the ice, where he or she is vulnerable to cuts from a skate blade. That's why good-quality equipment—gloves and neck guards especially—is a must. The goalie is also more likely to get a puck or stick in the head than other players. Having a good, well-fitted mask and helmet really cuts down on the risk. Of course, since the goalie regularly has shots being taken at him, there is an increased danger of concussion, but it's unlikely in the first few years.

And there will be bruises, despite all the protective gear. Treat them with Rest, Ice, Compression and Elevation (the R.I.C.E. principle), which I explain in Chapter 7, Hockey Health and Safety.

Although they're not skating all over the rink, goalies actually work harder than the other players. For one thing, they're on the ice for the whole game. They're flopping down, getting up, darting from side to side. Naturally, they get hot, and their extra equipment can trap body heat. So they're at risk of dehydration and need extra fluid during a game or practice. It is not uncommon to see goaltenders who keep a water bottle on the top of the net. Sometimes goalies spray the water over their face; personally, I'd rather see it going in the mouth, where it can be used by the body to regulate temperature.

Well, I've tried to give you a feel for what you need to know when your son or daughter says, "I want to play goal." Keep in mind that in the first few years it shouldn't be a big problem. First, the coach should be rotating kids through the position and, second, your hockey association will probably supply equipment. Remember that the quality of goal equipment and the relative slowness of the game in the early years mean that there's no more risk of injury than for the rest of the players.

That said, if your child shows talent, you have to decide how far you want to go. You can easily spend several hundred dollars on equipment every few years, although, as I've said, there are ways to keep the cost down.

The goalie is a key member of any team, and it takes a special person to play the position well. If your child is that kind of person, maybe you should give it a shot.

Pregame Equipment Checklist—Goalie

(The regular player checklist appears at the end of the previous chapter.)

Age: _____

Weight: _____

Height: _____

Usually, the league will supply goalie gear such as pads, gloves and stick.

____ Underwear	____ Goal pads	____ Hockey bag
____ Thin cotton socks	____ Chest and arm protector	
____ Jock/Jill	____ Neck guard	
____ Garter belt	____ Throat guard	
____ Skates	____ Trapper and blocker	
____ Skate guards	____ Goal stick	

____ Hockey socks (both garter belt and socks are optional; many goalies prefer just to wear their underwear beneath the pads)

____ Hockey pants (older players will use goalie pants)

____ Helmet/Facemask (player style is adequate for first few years)

____ Mouth guard (mandatory in U.S.A. from Peewee up)

Extras

Keep these extra items in the hockey bag; it could save you a lot of hassle: extra underwear, extra socks, tape (black, white and clear), skate hone, skate towel, laces, screwdriver, extra screws for the helmet and mask, water bottle, spare toe strap, asthma medicine if it's needed, and a puck and a tennis or hockey ball in case your goalie suddenly feels like stopping a few shots.

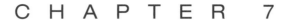

Hockey Health and Safety

As you may have gathered by now, I'm a doctor as well as a hockey player, coach and fan. It probably won't surprise you to know that I have special training in sports medicine, a relatively new medical field. (In Canada, sports medicine doctors pass an exam set by the Canadian Academy of Sports Medicine; in the United States, they are affiliated either with the American College of Sports Medicine or the American Orthopedic Society for Sports Medicine.)

In this chapter, I talk about the kinds of minor injuries I see in kids and what you—as a parent and primary caregiver—can do to prevent and treat them. The good news is that serious injuries are very rare indeed in kids' hockey. But it should go without saying that anything much beyond a bruise or a blister should be treated by a doctor. This chapter is emphatically *not* a substitute for proper medical care.

I think most injuries can be prevented—either by proper equipment that's properly fitted, or by good coaching and good hockey habits. But, as in any sport, accidents do happen and it's important to

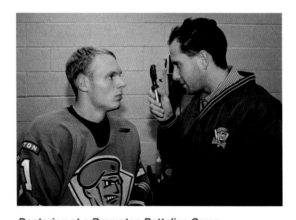

Doctoring at a Brampton Battalion Game

As team doctor for a Junior A hockey team, I see all sorts of injuries. But injuries are rare in the early years of hockey.

guard against them. I hate to hear about kids who got hurt and then decided that hockey was no fun. Our job as parents and organizers is to make sure they do have fun, in a safe, injury-free environment.

STRETCHING AND WARMING UP

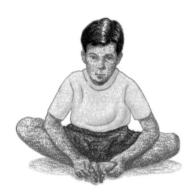

The Groin Stretch

Soles of the feet together, keep the back straight and press the knees toward the ground. You should feel the pull through the inner thigh.

Before playing any sport, players should warm up and stretch. And, yes, it's important for children, even young children, to stretch. Stretching temporarily lengthens a muscle and its attached tendons. Muscles that are well stretched are less prone to injury and can work better, which translates into better performance. Stretching also increases joint flexibility. For hockey players, stretching the legs is the most important, but the back and arms should not be neglected.

Often coaches will have the kids do a light warm-up by skating half-speed for a few minutes before stretching. Sometimes they don't call for any stretches. If you don't think the coach is having the kids do enough, have your child do some stretches at home before leaving for the rink. Don't be afraid to get on the floor and try them yourself. From among hundreds of stretches, I picked the ones illustrated here. Use them following these guidelines:

- Hold each stretch for a least 15 seconds.

- Do each stretch three or four times.

- If the stretch hurts, it's being done incorrectly.

If you can get your child to stretch every day for a few minutes, that's a good thing. Daily stretching keeps muscles loose and joints flexible. And even little kids can benefit from a daily regimen.

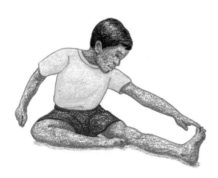

The Hamstring Stretch

Reach as far as you can toward the toes of the outstretched leg, keeping it as flat on the ground as possible. The other leg is folded to the side.

FITNESS FOR GOALIES

Goalies need to be more flexible than the other players, and they also have to develop muscle strength if they're to move those huge pads around quickly. Having your child simply wear the big pads around the house (if you own them or can borrow them) goes a long way to developing strength. To really improve, goalies need to work on increasing foot and reflex speeds. Sports such as soccer, tennis and racquetball are good for developing the right kind of hand-eye coordination for the position. Even juggling is an excellent way to develop goalie reflexes. Brian Daccord's book, *Hockey Goaltending*, shows some juggling exercises and has a great overview of goaltender fitness. (See Appendix 5.) Weight training, by the way, is not at all necessary.

There are three stretches I like for goalies: the sitting groin stretch, the quadricep stretch lying on the side, and the sitting hamstring stretch. The young goalie should perform these stretches as part of the warm-up in the dressing room.

One injury you hear about goalies getting more than other players is the groin pull. Sometimes the goalie will do the splits to make a save and slightly tear the groin muscles. Rest and physiotherapy are the only real treatments. Don't let your child go back in net if a groin injury isn't completely healed. A way to minimize the risk of this injury is to have the goalie work on doing the splits, but it may take months of *slow* practice before he or she can do them.

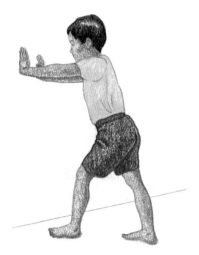

The Calf Stretch

Leaning against a wall, keep the head up and the back straight. One foot is closer to the wall than the other with both heels flat on the ground. You should feel the pull through the calf of the rear leg and the Achilles tendon.

STRENGTH TRAINING

Muscle strength plays a key role in preventing injury. Not that long ago, strength training for children was viewed as unsafe. Today, medical and fitness experts agree that strength training can be performed by children with very little risk of injury, as long as it's supervised and taught by people with proper training. Strength training means applying resistance to exercising muscles to make them stronger. Stronger muscles are less susceptible to injury and allow your child to perform better. Strength training is also used to recover from an injury.

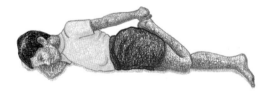

The Quadricep Stretch

Lie on your side with the head supported with the lower arm. With the other arm, grasp the foot of the upper leg and gently pull it toward the buttocks. You'll feel the pull through your thigh. Keep the back straight and the thigh in line with the body.

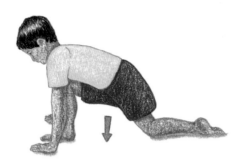

The Hip Flexor Stretch

Crouch down with the hands below the shoulders and one knee forward underneath the chest and the other leg extended behind with the knee on the ground. Push the hips toward the ground. Again, keep the back straight and the head up. You should feel a pull in the front of the hip (on the flexors). Make sure to switch legs.

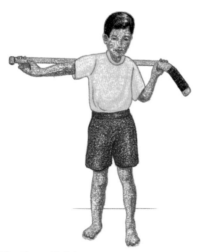

The Torso Twist

This dynamic (moving) stretch works the upper body and trunk. The hockey stick is placed across the shoulders and then rotated left and right with the upper body. Keep both feet firmly planted at shoulder width. Hold the stretch a few seconds at the end of each twist.

But strength training isn't weight training. It doesn't mean joining a gym or pumping iron. There are lots of fun exercises kids can do with a partner or by using their own body weight. One easy exercise is the standing long jump. The child sees how far he or she can jump from a standing position. Children can challenge each other or themselves as they try to increase their distance during the off-season. Piggyback races are fun, too. Hopping on one leg is a great way to develop strength *and* balance. I recommend a book called *Strength Training for Young Athletes* by Dr. William Kraemer and Dr. Stephen Fleck (see Appendix 5).

THE HOCKEY TRAINER AND MEDICAL HISTORY CARDS

Many teams have someone who acts as the trainer for the year. In fact, some hockey associations require that someone on the players' bench be designated as team trainer and have some type of certification. The trainer is responsible for managing any injuries that occur. Depending on the type of certification, the trainer may or may not have extensive first-aid and CPR training. (Cardiopulmonary arrest, by the way, is extremely rare in kids' hockey—an overexcited fan is more likely to require resuscitation than a player.) It's a good idea at the beginning of the season to check with the coach to see that there will always be someone with proper first-aid training (and an adequate first-aid kit) at practices and games. Keep in mind that, in general, rinks are not responsible for this function. Leagues and teams are.

The trainer usually keeps a medical history card for each player. The card lists allergies, asthma or any other medical condition a child may have and includes whatever medication he or she may be taking. On the card also appear your family's general practitioner's name and phone number, insurance information and an emergency contact number. These cards are important, particularly if another parent brings your child to the game.

In the United States, the National Sports Training Program was set up in 1997 to teach coaches how to prevent athletic injuries in children. There is also a Sport First Aid Course given by the American Sports Education Program (see Appendix 5). However, USA Hockey does not offer or arrange for any trainer courses, nor are there specific rules regarding a trainer being on the bench.

In Canada, the provinces offer Hockey Trainers Certification Programs. If you think you'd like to help out on the bench, this is one way. The programs usually run before the start of the hockey season, and you can sign up for one through your local association (see Appendix 5).

SPECIFIC INJURIES AND ILLNESSES

Blisters

Every year, at my hockey school, I treat several huge blisters. They are perhaps the most common injury kids suffer. They're caused by friction between the foot and an improperly fitted skate. As you'll have gathered from my discussion of skates (in Chapters 4 and 5), blisters are completely avoidable. If you haven't read those sections yet, check them out—you'll save yourself and your child a lot of grief.

But suppose a blister does develop? If it's small, leave it alone. Let it break on its own, if it's going to. If it's a large blister, break it with a sterilized needle. Boil the needle and then pierce the blister on the side to allow the fluid to escape. Leave the dead skin over top to protect the new skin underneath. Apply some topical antibiotic (Polysporin is a popular one) to the blister and cover it with a Band-Aid.

If the blister is large and painful, your child shouldn't skate until the foot can comfortably go back into the skate. To decrease friction, you might also put a small amount of Vaseline inside the skate, over the blister point.

Bruises and Contusions

Kids get bruises from running into each other, hitting the boards, falling on the ice, or taking a hit from a puck or stick on an unprotected area. The most common bruises occur on the front of the thigh (a charley horse), the outside of the arm, or the hip. (A hip bruise is usually called a hip pointer in hockey.) Technically, a bruise is the discoloration caused by bleeding into muscle or skin. It sounds worse than it usually is. A bruise on the shin, for example, is probably nothing to worry about. A charley horse, though, can be a problem because it may limit knee movement and delay a return to skating.

So, first aid for bruises? The R.I.C.E. principle of course. Rest. Ice. Compression. Elevation. (See below.) For simple bruises, you should have your child healthy again in no time. For pain, use acetaminophen (sold under various brand names, including Tylenol).

The R.I.C.E. Principle and Tensor Bandages

Bruises and contusions generally respond well to what I call the R.I.C.E. principle. Rest. Ice. Compression. Elevation. So do sprains and strains (I discuss them next). The R.I.C.E. principle makes for good first aid, but it's not a substitute for a doctor if you're worried or if the injury seems at all serious.

In general, rest is always a good idea, because movement can increase the bleeding or discomfort around an injured area. Apply ice every four hours, for about 10 minutes at a time. Crush some ice in a plastic bag (or use a bag of frozen peas), put it over the injured area (be it a bruise or a sprained ankle) and use a tensor bandage to hold it in place. A cloth or towel can act as a buffer between ice and skin. (Applying heat, by the way, is a bad idea. It will increase blood flow at exactly the time you want to slow it down.) The tensor bandage compresses the injured area, preventing more bleeding or swelling. And if you can manage to elevate the injured body part, you've got all four elements of the R.I.C.E. principle.

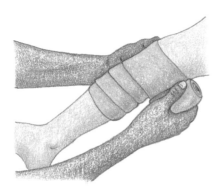

Applying a Tensor Bandage

Start below the injured area and work up. Overlap the previous turn by half to get a snug fit (but don't cut off the circulation).

So, tensor bandages compress and support an injured area. The compression limits swelling, which reduces pain and speeds healing. Tensors can help with some bruises. They're also good for an injury like a sprained ankle or a strained (torn) hamstring because they help to limit the movement of the injured joint and minimize pain.

Tensor bandages come in different sizes. For a child, a bandage two or three inches wide is appropriate. When you apply a tensor bandage, start below the injured area, to force any swelling up the injured limb. As you wrap the bandage, overlap the previous turn by half and give a little tug (not too hard!) to ensure a snug fit.

If, when you're done, there's swelling *below* the bandage, then you wrapped it too tightly. It's also too tight if your child complains that it hurts.

Sprains and Strains

A sprain is an injury to a ligament, the tissue that holds bones together at the joints. A strain is an injury to muscle or tendon. The best way to prevent both strains and sprains is through proper stretching. (See the first section in this chapter.)

Sprains aren't common in young kids, mainly because broken bones rather than injured ligaments tend to result from extreme pressure. But sprains do happen, and as a child grows up they become a more likely outcome of an accident than a break. Taking care of a sprain again involves the R.I.C.E. principle—Rest, Ice, Compression and Elevation (see above). But a joint injury is more serious than a bruise. Consult a doctor about management of the injury. And don't let the child back on the ice without the doctor's OK.

Tendons connect muscle to bone. A tear in the tendon or muscle—a strain—can be very painful. If the strain is bad enough, you may actually see bruising on the skin above the torn muscle or tendon. If you suspect a strain, see a doctor.

Fractures or Breaks

A broken bone (or a fractured bone—same thing) is going to put a cramp in your child's hockey playing for at least four weeks. Luckily, fractures are rare in kids' hockey. Kids are more likely to break a bone in the playground at school or on the ski slopes than on the ice. The most common fractures in kids' hockey occur at the wrist and the collarbone. As a rule of thumb, a collarbone injury will keep kids out for between four and six weeks, while a wrist fracture puts them off ice for between six and eight weeks. Depending on severity, those times can vary.

As a doctor, I often get asked about playing casts. My answer is that there is no such thing—especially at this level. For pros, with millions of dollars at stake, it may make economic sense (but not medical sense) to wear some sort of device that allows a return to action before the injury is completely healed. But a child should never return to hockey until the injury is healed and a doctor has given the OK.

Knee Pain

Lots of kids have knee pain. As a sports doctor it's one of the most common things I see in kids and adolescents. There are many causes, but the most common is irritation under the kneecap. Usually, it's nothing serious and the child will outgrow it. But—like a toothache or a migraine—it can make playing hockey no fun at all.

But if the knee pain seems serious or it looks as if there might be a problem with the joint, don't hesitate discussing it with your doctor. Some types of knee pain simply disappear over time—they're like a growing pain—while others respond very well to a simple, elasticized knee brace. A sports doctor can easily recognize a serious knee problem, and specialized braces for different kinds of knee pain are widely available.

Basically, knee pain should not prevent your child from playing any sport.

Head Injuries

Head injuries are uncommon in kids' hockey, because helmets protect against direct blows. So hitting the ice or the boards with the head is less of a danger than it used to be. On the other hand, helmets do *not* prevent the kinds of whiplash injuries that can shake the brain back and forth inside the skull, causing a concussion.

Doctors grade concussions on a scale of 1 to 3, with 3 being the most serious. That said, any concussion is cause for concern. Even the ringing sensation after a collision or blow to the head—what used to be called "having your bell rung"—should be taken seriously, although that would usually be diagnosed as a grade 1 concussion. If—and I stress this is unlikely—a player is knocked out during a game, he or she should not be moved and officials should call an ambulance. (The big worry here is a neck injury, about which more shortly.)

A child who is concussed should not play. That's flat. And if there's a suspicion that a child is concussed, he or she should be pulled out of the game or practice and taken to a doctor as soon as possible. Finally, a child should never return to sports until all symptoms from the head injury—such as headache, fatigue, dizziness and impaired concentration or memory—have resolved.

Neck Injuries

This is the big one—the type of injury that all parents fear, not only in hockey, but in any sport. Fortunately, with young children, neck injuries are rare. They do become more common as players get older and stronger. Remember: a helmet does *not* protect against neck injury. What does protect is knowing how to play the game safely. Education in safe play must begin from day one. Your child must learn to keep his or her head up at all times and never to hit another player from behind. Not many professional hockey players suffer neck injuries—they know how to protect themselves.

Classically, a neck injury occurs when a player is hit from behind, flies into the boards and hits the top of the helmet against the boards with the neck bent forward.

The same thing can happen without a dirty hit—kids can simply lose control and go flying into the boards head-first. (That's why learning to stop and turn properly is important; see Chapter 3 on basic skills.)

The best defense against illegal checks is education and enforcement. Kids have to know the possible consequences of a hit from behind. And referees and coaches should have zero tolerance. The best defenses against accidents are good skating skills and a habit of keeping the head up, not bent forward. (See the section on Body Contact and Checking in Chapter 3.)

The Common Cold

The common cold is caused by viruses that affect all children at one time or another. We can prevent colds, to some degree, by not sharing water bottles and by staying away from sick players. In my view, kids who are too sick to play should be kept away from the dressing room.

When I'm coaching, if I'm not sure whether a player is too sick to play, I use the Neck Check to decide. It's a simple principle: If the symptoms are below the neck, avoid intense activity. So, for instance, generalized aches, cough, fever, chills, vomiting and diarrhea are signs that playing hockey is out. On the other hand, if the symptoms are above the neck—stuffy or runny nose, mild sore throat or sneezing—then it is generally OK to play.

Any kind of fever rules out hockey. Exercise increases the core body temperature, and the combination of fever and the excess heat from exercise could lead to heat exhaustion. Rest, fluids and acetaminophen (e.g., Tylenol) for fever, aches and pains are the best medicines. Decongestants are also useful—but check with your family physician.

Returning after an Injury or Illness

Don't let your child go right into a game after returning from an injury. A practice is a better bet, or, if your child's team doesn't have practices, go public skating.

Why? Because these more controlled environments allow you to get an idea of how well the injury or illness has been overcome. As a general rule, players should be able to walk around easily, run and turn with no difficulties. After an injury, joint mobility and muscle strength must be restored gradually.

Asthma and Allergies

About one in every ten kids has asthma, a disease of the lung that results in swelling and narrowing of airways. If your child suffers from recurrent wheezing and coughing, he or she may have asthma. The first thing, if you suspect your child has asthma, is to see a doctor for an exam and lung function tests. Make sure, one way or another.

If the doctor says asthma is the cause of your child's wheezing and coughing, does this rule out hockey? Absolutely not. My eldest son, Brayden, has asthma and is turning into a fine young player who can skate like the wind. Indeed, many professional players have asthma. The key is managing the condition so it doesn't interfere.

If you or your child has asthma, you probably already know that asthma attacks can be triggered by colds, irritants like cigarette smoke, allergies to things like dust mites or grasses, cold air (in places like hockey rinks) and exercise. Since hockey is a form of exercise taken in cold air, the game can trigger an asthma attack. But if your asthmatic child is not having any symptoms while actually playing hockey, continue with whatever treatment your doctor has recommended. If your child is not using a device called an aerochamber, which helps more medication get directly into the lungs, ask your doctor to prescribe one. It attaches to the standard inhaler or puffer, which is less efficient on its own.

If your child is coughing, wheezing or more short of breath than the other children, he or she needs medication before, and possibly during, hockey games or practices. Most sports medicine doctors would recommend one or two puffs of a bronchodilater (a medication that opens up airways) 10 or 15 minutes before hockey or exercise. Keep extra medication in the hockey bag, just in case. And do make sure the coaches know about the problem and have been made aware of what symptoms to look out for. If the symptoms are severe and sometimes come on quickly, you may want to make sure your child takes medication to the bench.

If your child has an allergy, particularly if it's a food allergy (peanut butter is now a common one), let the coach know and inform the other parents. They need to know because often moms will make cupcakes or other goodies for the team if it's someone's birthday or the team is playing in a tournament. It's important that a child isn't inadvertently given something to eat that could do harm.

NUTRITION AND FLUID MANAGEMENT

Food and fluids are the fuel we use to keep active. Kids involved in a sport—especially a fast-paced, high-energy sport like hockey—need extra calories and fluids.

Keep it simple—avoid the snack bar at the rink (as much as you can!) and follow a well-balanced diet of carbohydrates, fat, protein, electrolytes (salts) and fluid. A pregame meal should be high in carbohydrates (fruits, vegetables and grains) and low in fat (meat and fast foods). Many of the Junior players I know like to eat a meal of chicken (it's low in fat if the skin has been removed and it wasn't deep fried) and pasta (high in carbohydrates) before a game.

Try to leave at least two hours between the meal and the game or practice; the child will be more comfortable on a relatively empty stomach. (I once saw a child vomit on the ice—it was the junk food dinner his parents bought him at the rink just before a game.) Remember, exercise interferes with the body's ability to digest food because blood is shunted to the working muscles and to the skin to cool the body.

After exercise, it's a different story. The muscles require refueling. This is a great time for a piece of fruit or a sport bar. That said, I know it's hard to keep the kids away from the concession counter. But common sense should prevail. A post-game treat, once in a while, is fine; don't get in the habit of dropping five bucks on junk food every time you come to the rink. It's a lousy way to spend money for something that is better left on the shelf.

Sport drinks, which are expensive and high in sugar, are not necessary for your child. If your child is playing in a tournament and has multiple games, sport drinks might not be a bad idea. They were, after all, scientifically formulated to enhance absorption of necessary electrolytes (or salts) and carbohydrates into the bloodstream of high-performance athletes. However, despite great advertising, I don't think sport drinks are better than water. But I will admit that they're better than soda pop, which is basically sugar and water (and caffeine in the colas).

Fluids, though, are important. For exercise lasting less than an hour, plain water is best. A good rule of thumb is between two and four ounces of fluid for every 15 minutes of exercise. So, in a sport like hockey, it is more important to have water available for practices or at a hockey school than during games, because in a game your child may get only 10 or 15 minutes of ice time. Half an hour or so before a game or practice, it's a good idea to have a cup of water.

> **TIP** Kids should *not* share water bottles. They are notorious for harboring germs and spreading infection. Every child should have his or her own water bottle—with a name on it.

And as a final note to this chapter, once it's on, hockey equipment can be fairly cumbersome to take off. Remind your child to go to the bathroom before getting changed.

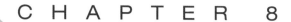

Good Hockey Parenting

Hockey is meant to be fun. Being a good hockey parent means keeping the fun in the game. The mission statement of the Canadian Hockey Association goes a long way to putting into perspective just what's important in kids' hockey. "We dedicate ourselves to the advancement of amateur hockey for all individuals through progressive leadership by ensuring meaningful opportunities and enjoyable experiences in a safe sportsman-like environment." It's that simple—and that complicated. Remember that playing hockey, or any sport, benefits children most when they can have fun while they do it. Over-competitiveness can be a big problem. Some parents get caught up in it and so do some coaches. But it's the young players who end up getting pressured and affected by those adults who sometimes simply need to take a step back. Keep that in mind when you're at the rink.

TIPS ON HAVING FUN AND SETTING GOALS

But what does all that mean exactly? Well, as a coach of many years I think I've seen what works and what doesn't. My heart goes out to those little players who just want to have fun on the ice while somebody—usually a parent—won't let them. Here are some things you should and shouldn't do.

Don't emphasize winning and competition. No team wins all the time, and your child is bound to wind up feeling miserable if he or she thinks winning is the only reason to play the game. The deeper and more widely spread benefit of sports comes not from winning but in developing social and physical skills. These contribute to a positive self-image. The main reason kids should play a sport is to have fun. In the first year or two kids really don't care about winning or losing. You'll see that for yourself if you go into the losing team's dressing room at the Novice level. There are no long faces—just happy, noisy children. Most players (even at the Junior level!) would much rather be on the ice for a losing team then sit on the bench of a winning team. Putting an emphasis on winning is a sure sign of a bad hockey parent.

Don't compare your child to the others. Comparison destroys fun. And it doesn't matter if it's positive or negative. Telling a player he's great but the rest of the team is awful is just as bad as the reverse. It doesn't hurt to compliment all the kids. After all, they are a team.

Do encourage, not criticize. Find at least one positive thing to say to your child after the game. And be specific: "That was a nice pass you made to your center when she was open in front of the net." Don't bother telling the player where he or she went wrong. It will either go in one ear and out the other or it will just squash your kid's enthusiasm. If you've seen a Beginner level game, then you know that in terms of pure hockey a lot more is going wrong than right. But the goals here are learning and fun. If your child makes a mistake, try to see the humor in it. It isn't the end of the world if your child trips over the blue line or takes a shot at his or her own net. (Believe me, it happens.)

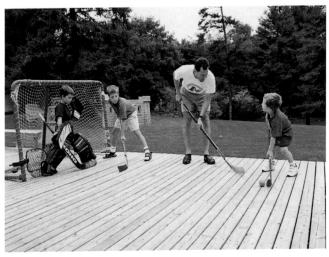

Me and the Kids
Here I am playing shinny with the kids. Of course, Spencer is in net.

Do get involved. Show up for the games, ask questions about the practices, even get out in the street and play a little road hockey (or shinny)—it shows your child that you can find the time to pay attention. And that means, in the child's mind, that he or she is important. So remember, hockey isn't just a baby-sitting service. Be there.

Do set goals. As you may have gathered, I don't like too much competition in kids' hockey, but there's nothing to stop you setting goals with your child. For instance, you might ask him or her to take more shots, or try to pass more, or learn to stop both ways. The goals don't have to be worked at only in the rink. With a sheet of plastic ice, your child can practice stick-handling, wrist shots and backhands in the basement or the garage. You can practice passing together on the driveway with a tennis or hockey ball or a foam puck. To me, those are healthy goals—and most importantly they're under the child's control. Skill development is part of building a child's self-esteem. Winning is not.

BEING A RESPONSIBLE PLAYER

When children join that first team, suddenly they belong to something bigger than anything they may have been part of before. The league and the coaches and the trainers all have their responsibilities to the team and the welfare of the players. But what about the young players' responsibilities? As the first year progresses and then the second, you'll see improvements happening all the time. But it isn't magic. Kids need to show up not just for the games, but for the practices too. They owe it to themselves and the team. So, here are a couple more tips.

Do emphasize commitment. Playing hockey means being part of a team. Once the child commits to the team, it's important to enforce that commitment—even if it means missing a birthday party or a television show. That said, there may be some exceptional circumstances, and it's up to you to judge when the child is physically or emotionally not ready to play.

Do show up on time. Sometimes lateness is a parent's fault and sometimes it's the player's fault. Either way, punctuality is a good virtue to instill. Being on time can really add to your child's hockey experience. Kids enjoy the time in the dressing room to fool around a bit and talk it up with teammates and coaches. Retired players have told me that the greatest part of the game was in the dressing room before and after the game.

Do check the equipment before leaving home. Use the checklists at the ends of chapters 5 and 6, if you like. A good habit for your child to get into is to check the equipment before leaving home. (Do oversee the checking, however.) You can avoid a lot of complications if you've ensured that everything needed for a game or practice is in the bag. It also really helps to have the equipment well maintained—skates sharpened, stick taped.

VACATIONS AND GROUNDING

I just finished talking about your child's commitment and responsibility to the team. As important as that may be, we shouldn't forget that the most important "team" in a child's life is his or her family. Sometimes family activities can take precedence over a child's sports activities. Family vacations are an example of this. If possible, try not to plan those winter vacations (if you can afford such things) during the season. If the child really loves hockey and has to miss a big game or a tournament, it may feel as if he or she is letting down the rest of the team. Each team usually has 15 players and can manage fine if a player or two are absent, but if your plans recurrently keep your kid away from games and practices, it might be time to think about scaling back some of those other activities. The coach, of course, deserves to be informed of any plans that keep a player away.

We all make mistakes, and sometimes a child makes a mistake that as a parent you feel warrants punishment. You may decide to withdraw extra-curricular activities from your child. That's your prerogative, but I'd suggest withdrawing game privileges and have your child continue with practices. Children's skills develop most through practices where they're on the ice all the time, rather than in games where they may see only 10 minutes of ice time in each match. Withdrawing a game or two sends a message, and keeping up with practices allows the child to increase his or her skill level along with the rest of the team.

BEING A RESPONSIBLE PARENT

Parents can become very excited at games. Sometimes it brings out the worst in people. I really urge you to be aware of how you behave in the rink. It's in your power to set an example for your own child and even other parents. Make it a good one.

Don't yell at the referee. Children learn from our actions, and this is a terrible thing to learn. Remember, it's pointless telling the child to respect the referees if you're up in the stands shouting abuse. You are the most important role model for your child. Think about it—eventually you might be the authority figure your child is yelling at.

Don't coach from the stands. Cheer your child on. But don't give orders—"Shoot!" "Pass!"—from the stands. If you want to play table-top hockey, buy a set and play it at home. Don't try to do it at the rink, with your son or daughter as a puppet. Try shouting "Good Shot" or "Good effort," or "Nice work" or "Nice try."

Don't yell at the coach—before, during or after the game. Your child's coach is a volunteer donating a great deal of time to the team. While you shouldn't get in the coach's face, you do have to be prepared to confront problems. If you think something is seriously amiss, talk about it with the coach. You should approach this situation as calmly and respectfully as you'd hope someone else would who was telling you the same thing. Talk with the coach in a collected and pleasant manner; be prepared to listen. Give the coach a chance to explain his or her position—there may be good reasons behind some coaching decisions that haven't occurred to you. At that point, having heard the coach's position, it's not unreasonable to expect that he or she hear you out. The situation is much more likely to be resolved successfully and pleasantly if both parties treat each other respectfully and keep cool heads. By the way, it is a bad idea to confront the coach at a game or practice—there's too much else going on. Arrange a good time for a phone call, or meet for lunch to discuss your concerns.

THE COACH AND ICE TIME

The coach is a powerful role model for your child, and particularly at the beginning of the season it's perfectly in line for you to ask some questions. What are the coach's qualifications and experience? Why is the coach involved with the team? What goals has he or she set for the season?

I've coached hockey for five years, and every year I learn more about it. I've made my share of mistakes, and sometimes suggestions and criticisms from parents have helped to make me a better coach. So, as a coach, I can say I'm always ready to listen. However, from my years around the rink, I've learned that coaches listen a lot more if they're not immediately put into a defensive position. Keep it in mind.

Ice time is a big source of complaints. Ideally, every player, good or bad, should get roughly the same amount of ice time. Before going after the coach on this one, though, take a moment to reflect. Parents naturally notice their own child most. What may look like an eternity could be very close to what all the players are getting on the bench. If you're quite sure, then you have a legitimate concern.

Even on rep teams, unless it's a sudden-death overtime situation or the closing minutes of a very close game, I believe all the players should be treated equally. (Some rep coaches, however, don't share my view.) If you're not satisfied with how your child's team is being coached, you can always talk to the coach. If you're still not satisfied, you can take your concerns to the league executive committee or the convenor for your child's age group and apply to have your son or daughter switch to another rep team or have him or her play in house league.

"I DON'T WANT TO PLAY ANYMORE"

If your child wants to stop playing or feels reluctant to go to games and practices, the most important question to ask is why. Sometimes kids run into problems with other players or the coach. Listen closely.

Don't ignore your child's feelings. What may seem like rough-and-tumble cama-raderie to you may feel like bullying to a child. There may really be a bully on the team. Perhaps your child feels he or she isn't contributing enough to the team. Or getting enough ice time. Perhaps the coach, with the best will in the world, is scaring or alienating your young player. Listen closely.

Do ask other adults. You can try talking to the coach or assistant coach. Or the trainer. Maybe they've noticed something, too.

Do ask yourself, too. Did you push your child into hockey because of your own interest in the game? Is that why the child doesn't want to get up for those early-morning practices?

You may want to get extra instruction for your child if it seems like a confidence problem. (At minimum, you can always go public skating together.) If it seems the problem is really with the team or the coaches, you can request to change to another team. If the problem concerns the coach's behavior, verbal or physical, talk to your local association's convenor or another league official.

If your child really wants to stop playing after a little while, most leagues will at least partly refund registration fees. The equipment can be resold at an equipment exchange. But before you do that you might simply want to wait for next year and see if your child wants to play then. Much of the equipment will still fit and some of it can be traded up at equipment exchanges.

ABUSE

In the past few years there have been several high-profile cases of sexual abuse in hockey. Most involve coaches or officials of elite teams, whose players were away from home (and their parents' supervision) for long periods. These are horrifying to all real hockey fans, not just because they involved an enormous breach of trust, but because they destroyed the joy of the game (and much else) for several young men.

Let me emphasize that cases of sexual abuse in hockey are extremely rare. In the first years of hockey—where you and lots of other parents are in and out of the dress-ing room—and there's little or no traveling, I would go so far as to say there's almost no chance of sexual abuse.

That said, it's important to talk to your child about the issue. Tell him or her there are some places they shouldn't be touched by an adult. Make sure the commu-nication lines are open. Also, you should keep an eye open—watch how the child interacts with the coaches and players; be alert for unexplained bruises or marks, especially near the genitals; be especially wary if the child's behavior or demeanor changes markedly at hockey.

Sexual abuse isn't the only kind, of course. Physical and verbal abuse—bad language, unjust punishments, humiliation, to name just a few possibilities—are equally unwanted.

So what should you do? If it's something simple, like the occasional outburst of bad language, I'd just approach the offending coach and ask him or her to lay off. More serious problems call for professional help—either from social workers, doctors or the police. If you think something is seriously wrong, don't mess around. Get help.

COACHING AND ASSISTING

Very often coaches are involved because they have a child on the team. One thing leads to another, and they take a course. Then they find that they enjoy coaching and take even more courses. One way many parents start this process is by volunteering as an assistant coach. What this means, at the most basic level, is that you stand in the team bench and open the doors so the players can go on and off the ice. As an assistant coach, of course, you also tie skates, adjust equipment, deal with emotional crises ... all the pleasures of dealing with kids.

If you decide you like coaching, consider a formal course. The Canadian Hockey Association offers a one-day course called the Canadian Hockey Initiation Program, which teaches you some basics that you can pass on to kids between 5 and 9. The Association also offers more intensive courses that qualify you to instruct at a higher level. In the United States, USA Hockey has similar programs. In both countries, you can usually sign up through your local association. I've included more detailed information on becoming a coach in Appendix 3. (If you see yourself in stripes, both organizations also offer courses in how to become a referee. See Appendix 4 for more details.)

Being a coach is a challenge. The coach has to develop player skills, keep the game fun, make sure all the kids are treated fairly, and not be distracted by the all-too-obvious goal of winning. In today's all-or-nothing competitive society, that last one is especially hard. If you find that your son or daughter has landed on a team with great coaching, don't forget to thank those individuals.

SINGLE PARENTS

Many of you reading this book are single parents. It can be hard enough juggling children's activities with two parents; with just one it can be a huge challenge. If you have more than one child at home, it may seem like you're climbing Everest everyday. I've said that good hockey parents show up, but you obviously have other things you *must* do. Your child likely understands this; after all, he or she is part of the family and knows the stresses you're under. When you can't make it to a game or practice, often other parents offer to help out with rides. Informal car-pooling is almost as old as hockey itself. Some days you'll pick up one or two extra players, and on other days it will be a different parent who is helping you out. After all, they'll be at the rink themselves during the game or practice. Just remember that you shouldn't always be on the receiving end, and some day they'll need the favor returned. Your child will understand if you don't make it to all the games, but he or she will feel a lot better when you do. The message it sends is that your child is important.

The stresses on families today, whether single- or two-parent, are enormous. You may actually find the relative calm of the rink to be a relief. Bring the newspaper or a book to practices. If you need to tell someone how horrible you feel getting up so early, there'll be lots of other parents to talk to.

MY CHILD PLAYS GOAL

I'll just touch on this again here briefly since I've already discussed these issues in Chapter 6. Remember that it's a tough job, physically and mentally. Goalies especially should stretch before games. That aside, let me reiterate a few important aspects about the goalie.

The goalie sees a different game than the other players. While the rest of them are out scrambling for the puck or sitting on the bench, the goalie is watching everything on the ice, trying to be prepared for that next shot or breakaway that could come at any time. The mental focus and pressure are greater and more sustained. And even if a goalie plays a great game and makes 10 great stops and lots of little ones, the team might still lose—because of the one or two shots that got by. The goalie may feel individually responsible for a loss. It's very important to remind this player that the whole team wins or loses a game. You might remind him or her that the great Ken Dryden let in plenty of goals during his NHL career and his team certainly didn't win every game. It wasn't always winning that made Dryden a great player. It was always getting up after a victory or a defeat and saying, well, I think I can do better. (Dryden's book *The Game* is a great view of hockey from between the posts.) As a parent, you can always offer to practice taking shots on your young goalie at home.

FIGHTING AND CONFLICT RESOLUTION

What about fighting? I discuss this at length in Appendix 2, but for now let me state the most important points. As a parent you need to teach your aspiring hockey player that fighting is not right. How can you do this? I think you say that fighting is not tolerated in our society. We don't allow it in the playground or school. Consequently, it should not be allowed in a hockey rink.

If your child gets in a fight, the chances of physical injury are small. The part of the body most likely to get hurt is the hand of the child throwing a punch if he's dropped his gloves—but the referees are usually there long before that point in kids' hockey. The real damage comes if the incident isn't given proper attention. The player needs to understand that fighting is not an acceptable response to frustration or anger. Even if the ref didn't think it was a real fight and hands out only two-minute penalties, the coach should consider sitting the player out the rest of the game. How else can a child learn that fighting is not tolerated?

After the game, it's very important to sit down and find out why it happened. Hear the child out. Try to understand his or her point of view. Above all, don't make light of the issue. You are the key to your child's understanding of the game. An apology to the other player after the game isn't a bad idea either.

THE HOCKEY HALLS OF FAME

Hockey parenting isn't all finger wagging. It can be lots of fun, too. During the season or in the off-season, a visit to the Hockey Hall of Fame is a nice family activity if you can make it into Toronto, Ontario, or Eveleth, Minnesota.

In Toronto, the Hockey Hall of Fame officially opened in 1961 on the grounds of the Canadian National Exhibition. In 1993, the hall was moved to the heart of downtown Toronto, where it is housed in a hundred-year-old former bank building.

If you're in Toronto, take your family for a visit. The hall's exhibits—including a replica of the Montreal Canadiens' old dressing room at the (now-defunct) Forum—cover amateur and pro hockey for the past century. Early equipment, modern goalie masks, the Stanley Cup itself—it all combines to make a great outing for a hockey fan.

The Hall's American counterpart—the United States Hockey Hall of Fame—is in Eveleth, Minnesota. It opened in 1973, and in 1999 underwent a multimillion-dollar renovation. It has a host of features, including a spectacular memorial to the

1980 Miracle on Ice, when the United States Olympic team beat the heavily favored Soviet Union in Lake Placid. There's also a look at the United States women's hockey team that won the 1998 Olympic gold medal.

I give their addresses and telephone numbers in Appendix 5.

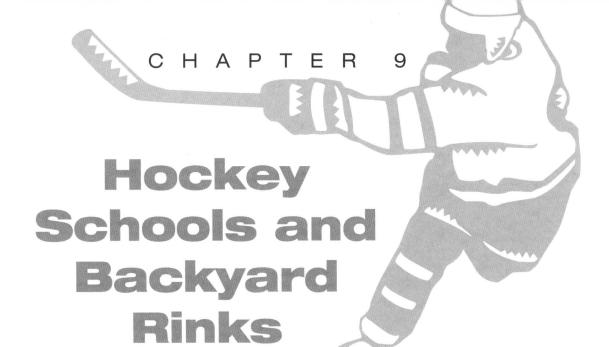

CHAPTER 9

Hockey Schools and Backyard Rinks

CHOOSING A HOCKEY SCHOOL

I played lots of hockey growing up—from Beginner to Midget. Even for my first few years of college I played for the University of Waterloo (Ontario) Warriors. But getting to that level wasn't simply a matter of one game and one practice a week. I spent a lot of time on the ice. I know now how lucky I was. My dad built a little rink in our backyard every winter, and in the summers I'd often go to a hockey school for at least a week or two. I look back on these things now and I realize how much they helped to instill a deep love of the game in me. I'm not saying that you need to provide these things to your child for him or her to enjoy hockey. In fact, some kids enjoy hockey more when it's an occasional (but regular) activity. But if hockey is your kid's number one pastime and he or she has a real craving for more ice time and better skills (and you can afford it), then knowing a little bit about choosing a hockey school can be a big help. And though knowing how to build a backyard rink may be more than you ever want to know about hockey, I've included instructions in case this book falls into the hands of some real enthusiasts.

To tell the truth, just plain ice time is a valuable thing in itself. Public skating is a great way to develop skills on the ice. Starting, stopping, turning can all improve with regular skating. Speed and confidence will improve, too. If you live where outdoor rinks and frozen ponds are available all winter, then a daily game of shinny with the other kids is one of the best ways for your child to improve his or her hockey skills—and have fun doing it. But these days, more and more families live in places where time on the ice, whether natural or artificial, is hard to come by. Hockey schools and camps are filling the gap.

If you think your child would benefit from more ice time, coupled with instruction, then a hockey school could be the answer. The question is how to pick a good one from the thousands that are available. I've been teaching children ages 6 to 12 every summer since 1982 at my Albion Hills Hockey School in Caledon, Ontario. I've also sent my two oldest boys to hockey schools other than my own. So over time I think I've learned what to look for in a hockey school. But let me state my biases first. Yes, learning hockey skills is important. But it should never come at the expense of the children having fun as they learn. It's a game.

Hockey schools used to run mostly in the summer, but you can now find them all year round. There are weekend hockey schools, those operating during school breaks, sleepaway camps during the summer and every possible combination of the above. Some specialize in kids with a certain skill level, age or position. Some schools focus on goal-scoring, some on checking, others on defense play or stick-handling or passing. Most are co-ed, but some are only for girls. There's plenty of choice. Let me caution you, though. If your child can't skate, then a hockey school is *not* appropriate. There are learn-to-skate programs in most communities, and that should be the first step.

So how to start? A good place is at the local rink, where brochures and advertisements can often be found. The staff may also have some ideas. The weekly paper *The Hockey News* usually publishes a guide to hockey schools in North America every January. If you know other parents with kids in hockey, ask for their recommendations. And don't be afraid to drop in to a school to check it out. The hockey school you choose will depend on your child, your schedule and your budget. But here are some things to think about as you make the decision.

First of all, budget. The good news is that most hockey schools have fees comparable to other types of specialty camps. Day camps are often very convenient and, of course, they're better for the very young kids, who'd feel lonely away from home. Overnight camps, on the other hand, offer the opportunity to try other sports, such as golf, tennis, boating and horseback riding, while keeping the emphasis on hockey.

Your child's welfare and safety are paramount, whichever kind of hockey school you choose. Here are a few guidelines to help you choose:

- Make sure the facility is in good operating condition and the ice surface is well maintained. Also make sure the facility is constructed so it is easy for counselors and instructors to supervise the children.

- Make sure the instructors and counselors have some first-aid and/or CPR training. They should have some type of emergency action plan.

- If you can, observe a few on-ice sessions to ensure the players are kept busy and are being provided with instruction. Be suspicious of any hockey school that does not welcome parents to observe.

- Also make sure the kids will be kept busy with off-ice activities. Most day camps organize games like baseball, soccer or ball hockey. At the camp I operate, I also like to use instructional videos during the off-ice time. I list some tapes in Appendix 5.

- Three hours of ice time a day is usually enough. Stay away from camps that advertise five and six hours of ice time; that's simply too much, and also a great way to turn your child off the sport.

- Typically, schools will group together players aged 6 to 9 and 10 to 12. Most schools will have between 20 and 30 skaters per session, and up to four goaltenders. A good student-to-instructor ratio is about seven to one.

- Most children under 9 cannot tighten their own skates; ensure the school has enough staff to help. The younger ones may also need help with their equipment.

- Many schools offer power skating, which is, simply put, teaching the proper stride and technique for playing hockey. You'll often find figure-skating coaches teaching power skating; they make excellent instructors because of the emphasis on skating in their sport. But power skating is not exactly fun; most kids think it's about as entertaining as eating brussels sprouts. If you've decided to enroll your child in power skating, do emphasize that skating is the most important skill in hockey.

- If your child is a goaltender, but is attending a school that has both players and goalies, make sure there is a goaltender instructor. You don't want your child used only as a target.

While it may seem that the hockey school or camp will relieve your hockey parenting responsibilities for at least a bit of time, you still play a key role, especially since most small children have no idea of how to get organized for a day (or a week) away from home. Here are some tips to help make hockey school easier on you and your child:

- Organize your child's equipment and make sure it all fits. If your child has already played last season, for example, I guarantee at least one piece of equipment will have been outgrown since then. Replace the outgrown stuff and check to make sure that the rest isn't showing too much wear. (See Chapter 4 for fitting guidelines.)

- If your child will need new skates, get them well in advance and try to break them in beforehand. Hockey schools are not the place to break in skates. (See Chapter 4 for guidelines on breaking in new skates.)

- Get the skates sharpened. You'll need to do it again every three to four days.

- Your child will probably need a new stick; most kids grow an inch over the summer. Make sure you put a name on it.

- In fact, label all equipment with your child's initials. Children are not usually neat when removing equipment, and when you have 15 or 20 kids in a room, things do go missing. Initials on equipment also come in handy for the counselors who are helping the kids get dressed.

- Sit down with your child and practice how to get dressed for hockey.

- Put an extra pair of laces in the hockey bag. There is nothing more frustrating than trying to tie up skates with frayed laces.

- If your child wears socks to play (some prefer bare feet in their skates), then put several dry pairs in the bag.

- Every night, dry out the equipment (you can usually just hang it up) and check for any missing items. Don't panic if something is missing; it is usually in some other child's bag, or an instructor has picked it up.

- If the child is asthmatic, make sure the inhaler goes to camp. Don't forget to tell the counselor.

- Pack a good lunch. Don't let your child buy lunch at the snack bar; I've seen what most kids will buy and eat! Children burn up lots of calories at camp; they need good nutrition. They will also need snacks throughout the day. Check if the hockey school provides any snacks or drinks as part of the package.

- For off-ice activities in summer, send shorts, a T-shirt, sunscreen, good running shoes (not sandals!) and a hat.

Overnight or "sleepaway" hockey camps deserve some special mention. All the above points apply, but there are some additional considerations:

- Find out about the training and responsibility of the camp counselors. Remember, these counselors essentially play the parental role during camp.

- Find out about the camp's medical coverage. If you're enrolling your child in a camp in another country, ensure there's proper medical insurance.

- Most schools will want to know your child's allergies and if he or she is on any type of medication. Make sure any medication goes with your child, and that the counselor knows schedules and doses.

Some schools advertise NHL players as part of the program. Make sure that the player is giving instruction, rather than just showing up, signing some autographs and then going home. Ten or 20 years ago, many NHL players earned extra money by working at or operating a hockey school. With today's astronomical salaries, NHLers no longer need the money. So they usually demand a fairly high fee for their services, making programs with NHL players more expensive.

Bear in mind that just because a player has made it to the NHL doesn't mean he will automatically relate well to kids and be able to teach them. I have operated a hockey school for over 15 years, and throughout those years I have used College- and Junior-level players, not NHLers. I do not necessarily seek out the best hockey player, but I look for the individual who relates well to the kids and can get down to their level. Pretty much any hockey player in the Junior or College ranks is fairly skilled and has more than enough knowledge to impart. The key is to be able to get it across.

A final note. After a week of hockey camp, don't expect your child to play like Wayne Gretzky. You'll see the greatest gains early on, when your child is a weaker player, but over the years the gains will be less dramatic. For some kids, the week of hockey camp may be the most ice time they've ever had and they'll blossom. More experienced players won't make the same leap. But, veteran or novice, if they learn one new concept or skill each day, then camp will have been a success. Becoming a hockey player is a slow, gradual process. The key is to get the ice time and keep it fun.

THE BACKYARD RINK: A LOST ART

I will always remember the hours I spent on the backyard rink my father built every winter. Our rink wasn't big, but to my young eyes it was Maple Leaf Gardens. The ice was always hard and fast. There were no shifts; I played the entire game. There was no whistle or clock to tell me when the game was over. I made up my own rules. There was no such thing as an icing or off-side. The only stoppage in play occurred when I was so hungry and cold I had to go in to warm up, have a quick bite, and then get back on the ice.

I have that in common with the greatest player to ever play the game, Wayne Gretzky, who practiced for hours on his backyard rink in Brantford, Ontario. The story goes that his father, Walter, built a backyard rink because he was tired of taking Wayne to a nearby park that had ice. With a rink in his yard, Walter could watch his children from the comfort of his kitchen. In my opinion, it was the hours Wayne spent on the Gretzky rink that allowed him to develop his incomparable skills.

My three sons, Brayden, Spencer and Bryce, learned how to skate on our backyard rink. To this day they prefer fooling around in the backyard to a regular practice or game. And when people ask me why my kids skate so well, I tell them it's nothing special—I just built the rink and they took it from there. They skate for hours every day and eventually everything just clicks. Kids don't need coaches and referees to play a game of hockey (or something like hockey). Many of the skill drills in this book, by the way, were designed by me with the limited ice space of a small ice surface in mind.

If you have the space (and, of course, the climate), a backyard rink can be a great resource for your child—and all the neighborhood kids. It's just a fun thing, and not really all that hard to do. In this section, I'll describe two ways to build a backyard rink.

The beautiful thing about a backyard rink is that it doesn't have to be big. The first rink I built was actually a front yard rink for my younger brother—about 15 feet by 20 at my parents' home. This is all the space a child needs to master basic skills: stopping, turning, puck control, and shooting. The rink at our own house is not much bigger, but it has room for three kids—and Dad, too.

You can't have natural ice until the temperature is consistently below 32 degrees Fahrenheit (0 degrees Celsius). In the northern United States and most of Canada, that probably means mid-December or later. But it's a good idea to do the planning early and to build your frame before the first snow.

You do need a reasonably level plot of land. If you have a really uneven section, you might need to plan even earlier—say, during the spring—and lay down some topsoil and plant some grass. A tree in the middle of the rink makes an excellent object for the kids to stick-handle around or use as a defense player.

Here are a few tips before you start:

- Try to build the rink in shade; it will last longer in the spring. You will have to be careful to make sure that leaves and other tree debris don't get frozen into the ice.

- Don't worry about damage to the grass; most of the time it comes back fine.

- The shape can be anything you like—round, square or, like mine, with one end bigger than the other.

Some people like to build full boards, but personally, I prefer just a low frame that stops the puck from sliding off the rink. (You have to think ahead. You'll be the one shoveling the snow off the ice. Do you really want to lift it over four-foot boards?)

I use 2 x 8 or 2 x10 lumber, cut to fit the perimeter of the planned rink. Your lumberyard will cut it to suit you.

I put the boards end to end and nail wooden braces over the joints to keep them together. Use galvanized nails to prevent rust and don't drive the nails all the way in—that way disassembly will be easy. You can also use snow packed along the outside of the boards to help hold them together. The end result is a low 8- or 10-inch-high container for the water you'll shortly be spraying.

Many people swear by the following method. I've tried it. It works. But I like to add another wrinkle, which I'll tell you about in a minute. Meanwhile, here's the old-fashioned approach:

1. Wait until the ground is frozen and covered with a few inches of snow. Then compact the snow, either by trampling it or by using something like a heavy garden roller.

2. If you have built a frame, you work only on the snow inside it, of course. Otherwise, be sure to leave a border of higher snow to contain the water.

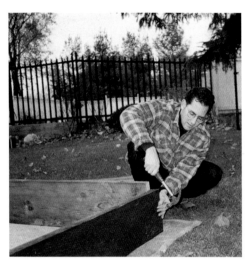

The Backyard Rink
Make the corners first, then join them up with the remaining boards.

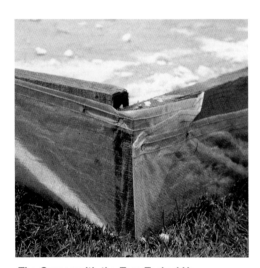

The Corner with the Tarp Tacked Up
Use galvanized shingling nails or staples to tack the tarp up all around.

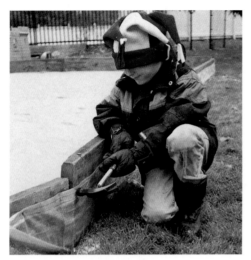

Brayden Helping with the Rink
Your child might like to help build the rink—as Brayden (age 7) does here.

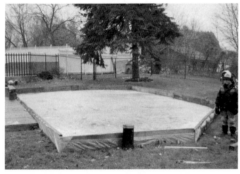

The Finished Product
Now it's just a matter of waiting for a cold snap.

3. Finally, you can start your first spraying of water on the compacted snow to let it turn to ice.

Simple, huh? Well, there are a few things to watch for:

1. For the first layer, sprinkle the water gently with a soft spray from a garden nozzle. And not too much—if you melt the snow underneath, the water will just be absorbed into the ground.

2. Don't use the outside tap—it will probably be frozen. You're better off to buy a tap adapter and run a hose through a window from the kitchen or basement sink. Do remember to take the hose in for the night; if it freezes, it's not easy to get it thawed.

3. Try not to let leaves or other debris get caught in the ice. They can interfere with skating if they're near the surface, and even if they're covered they can absorb sunlight and weaken the ice near them.

4. Depending how cold it is, you can usually put down a new coat of water every hour or so. Be patient. You need many coats of ice before the rink will be ready for skating.

5. About four inches of ice is enough for skating. Any thinner, though, and you risk losing the rink when the first warm snap hits.

Here's the wrinkle I call the bathtub method:

1. Once you know what size you plan to make the rink, get a heavy-duty plastic tarpaulin that's just slightly bigger overall. (Thin plastic won't work; it can't take the weight of the water and it tears.) A tarp custom-made to my specifications (by a local company) cost me about $100 and I reuse it every year. Get clear plastic. Black or colored plastic will absorb sunlight and speed melting in the spring. If you can get it with grommets around the edges, even better.

2. Now build the corners of your rink as I described above, nailing them together with galvanized nails. Lay out the tarp where you plan to build the rink. Put the prebuilt corners on, each in its place, to hold down the tarp.

3. Finally, join up the corners with the remaining boards.

4. You should now have the frame sitting on the tarp, with about six inches of plastic sticking out all around. Tack the plastic up on the *outside* of the frame. If you have grommets you can drive large-headed roofing nails into the frame to hold the plastic tarp in place. You can also use shingle nails or a stapling gun if there are no grommets. Whatever method you use, keep in mind that you'll have to take the nails or staples out in the spring. Fill the "tub" with water and wait for freezing temperatures.

5. Disassembly is dead easy. Take out the shingle nails or the staples that held the tarp to the boards. Then knock down some of the boards to let the melted water drain. Take the nails out of the wood and store it away. (I label the boards so I know which is which for next winter.) Give the tarp a wash, and after it's dry fold it up and put it away.

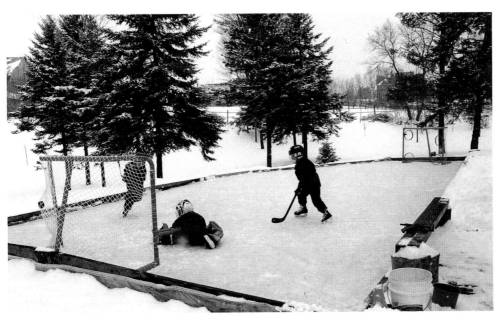

My Kids Playing on Our Backyard Rink
Winter's here!

The advantage of the bathtub method is that you don't have to wait for snow—just cold weather. And, you don't have to worry too much if there's a slight incline on your property. At home, we wind up with about a foot of ice at one end and six inches at the other.

With both types of rink, you need to keep the snow off, which means getting out the shovel. And it's probably a good idea to scrape the ice and flood it after the rink has been used—which at my house means every night! (Just a thin coat of water is all you need.)

Toward the spring, the ice can melt near the boards, creating gaps that can be dangerous. Fill these gaps with some snow and then sprinkle with water; you don't want a skate blade getting caught.

The backyard rink is a great hockey tradition. At our house, we put some lights outside so we can skate at night. At Christmas, it's a wonderful sight with lights dangling in the trees and around the rink. I have also built a little fireplace for the kids to warm their toes and hands when they take a break. And for the parents, the rink isn't just a chore. My wife or I often go for a skate or play a little shinny with the kids (if they'll let us on instead of their friends), and we don't need to drive the boys to other ice rinks or arenas to skate. My rink—I should say our rink—is great fun. If you try it, I bet you'll say the same.

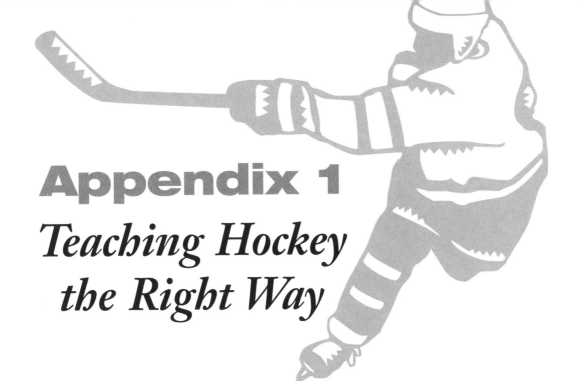

Appendix 1
Teaching Hockey the Right Way

I have a simple view of teaching hockey: Give the kids a puck and some ice, and let them have fun. I'm not a big fan of competition in children's hockey. I *am* a big fan of creativity in hockey. In my view, the European approach—with its creative and fun emphasis on skating and puck-handling—is the right way to go. This is why we are seeing professionals from Europe take elite roles in the National Hockey League. (About 65 percent of all the players are Canadians.) In 1999, Finnish player Teemu Selanne of the Anaheim Mighty Ducks won the Maurice "Rocket" Richard trophy for most goals scored. In fact, Canadians—once the most skilled—have become merely the goons and role-players (that is, checkers or penalty killers, not goal-scorers or finesse players) of the NHL. What has changed since the 1950s and 1960s, when Canada produced dozens of top-notch skilled players? I think back then players learned their skills playing shinny—no clocks, no refs, no face-offs—and only later graduated to organized hockey.

As major a figure as Wayne Gretzky—a wizard on ice for decades—has called for more fun and creativity in hockey. He summed up his participation in the 1999 Hockey Summit in Toronto with these words: "My big thing is we need to get back some creativity for youngsters." You may find the word creativity unusual in this context. Isn't hockey all about large men, with sticks in their hands and blades on their feet, bashing each other senseless? Well, no, not really. When it's played well, by truly skilled players, it requires breathtakingly fast thinking and stellar physical skills, with no room for error. But to achieve that level, we must encourage our kids to use their imagination, to unleash their physical and mental skills. And the first step is teaching those skills.

Hockey is a game of skating, puck control and thinking. Too often, a kids' game today resembles nothing more than glorified Ping-Pong. The puck is a hot potato, with a gang of kids chasing it. When one child does come up with the puck, too often he or she can't control it well enough to do anything useful. The basic skills of hockey are becoming a lost art.

Why? I think it is because the game today is too organized. The kids start playing games, with all those complicated rules, before they've mastered the basic skills. And yet it's at this young age when a very little instruction goes a very long way. At 6 and 7, kids' skills develop at an amazing pace if they're guided, taught and—a key point—allowed to play with the puck.

In my hometown house league, I introduced what may seem like a radical concept. For the 7-year-olds, we dropped the off-side and icing rules (see Chapter 2) and didn't bother with face-offs after goals were scored. (As in pickup hockey, the team that was scored on just took the puck back up the ice and tried to score in its turn.) It was an enormous success. We didn't waste time lining up for face-offs and blowing whistles. Instead the kids got to skate and play with the puck, and the parents sat back and watched the fun.

Another thing: Because we put so much emphasis on winning and losing, on competition in general, we jam children into slots. I hate to see coaches say, "So-and-so is slow; she'll play defense." Once they've assigned a position to a kid, that child is almost forbidden to break out. Heaven forbid that a defense player should attack. To put it simply, kids should be playing different positions.

But many coaches slot kids into one position and then try to teach "systems" or specialized plays to the children in the belief that using these systems (or "team tactics") gives them a better chance of winning. Jason Spezza, a talented youngster who played for the Brampton Battalion Junior A team, said this of his experience in youth hockey: "We worked on systems, we didn't work on finesse skills. We had to work on that ourselves." What he was learning from his coaches were plays and positional hockey—useful tools, but not important to children's hockey. To work on the necessary basic skills, Jason said, he took power-skating courses and practiced shooting in the basement with his little brother.

In this book I did not talk about systems or team tactics because I see little role for them in children's hockey. There's no point in introducing complicated systems (like a power play or neutral zone trap) if the basic skills (like passing and stickhandling) are not mastered. Today, there is some movement away from this "systems" approach to coaching, but there's still a lot of opposition, particularly at the rep and select levels.

Another problem I see in children's hockey today is that kids play far too many games and don't practice enough. In a typical game, a player will get 10 minutes of ice time, may touch the puck six times, get one or two shots on goal and possibly stick-handle the puck for 30 seconds. The weaker players may not even touch the puck. Think about what this means. In a 50-game schedule, the child gets 500 minutes of ice time, possibly 100 shots on net and 25 minutes of stick-handling. Kids could get all that in a weekend if they had access to a frozen pond or a backyard rink. Imagine a winter's worth of weekends like that. How well would your child skate and handle the puck?

A more recent prescription (which I agree with) is more practice, but many parents and coaches say, "Where's the fun in that?" Well, at my practices, we have lots of fun. Why? Because I focus on simulating game situations which involve skating, passing and shooting. For instance, I often have the kids playing a three-on-three game, so they have lots of space to try out new moves and lots of chances to get and control the puck. Or I let the kids play hockey with a soccer ball—but without sticks. Sometimes we play the grand old game of British bulldog, where a couple of players are in the middle of the ice and the rest of the team tries to skate past without being touched. Like the soccer ball game, it's great for balance and agility. Even though it looks like only fun and games to the parents and kids, the players *are* learning basic skills.

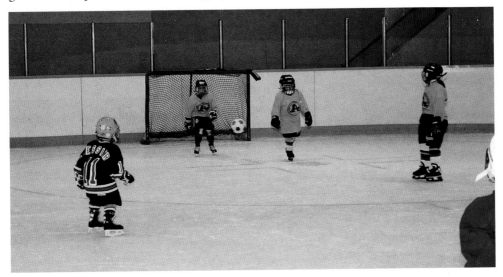

Kids at My Hockey School
Imaginative exercises—like a game of soccer hockey—can make practices fun, while teaching fundamental physical skills.

Some parents and organizers think that a game is better than a practice because it puts two teams on the ice. That's true, but only 12 of the 30-odd kids are on the ice at any one time—and half the time is wasted with stoppages in play. With ice time in such short supply, I think we need to make better use of what little time is available. For practices, two teams could practice at once— there's more than enough room for 30 kids on the ice. Further, several mini games could be played simultaneously across the ice instead of only one played end to end. Children will develop their skills much quicker with more practices and fewer games. And as I said above, it's easy to make practices fun for the kids.

I also believe that today in kids' hockey the season is just too long. In all-star or rep hockey, the games and practices start in August and go into March. Then parents put their kids into a succession of hockey schools for the summer. Now, I own and operate a hockey school. I think hockey schools have a role to play. But let's give the kids a break—let them play soccer or baseball or learn gymnastics. These other sports develop skills that complement hockey; playing catcher for a baseball team is great training for a goalie, for instance. And let's not forget that many of hockey's greats— such as Gordie Howe or Wayne Gretzky—were all-round athletes.

Kids who play hockey all summer are sick of it and burned out by Christmas. I see 12-year-old kids in my sports medicine practice who have played hockey all year-round for several years. The parents wonder why the child is developing muscle aches and pains. I explain to them that even professionals in the NHL take the summer off. In fact, the professional players' association, the NHLPA, mandates the maximum length of time players can play and practice. They do this because they realize players are susceptible to injuries and fatigue—both of which affect their livelihood.

For children's hockey, USA Hockey and the Canadian Hockey Association are primarily responsible for regulating the game in North America. These organizations do an excellent job of overseeing the rules and ensuring that kids can play hockey in fun, safe environments. Many conscientious and concerned individuals are part of USA Hockey and the CHA, and much thought goes into the almost constant review of their policies and philosophies. This is necessary because the game is constantly changing. Not surprisingly, however, such large organizations sometimes have difficulty keeping up with the pace of change at the grassroots level. While I am personally grateful for the role that the CHA has played in providing me (when I was a child) and my own children with opportunities to play the game, I feel that sometimes USA Hockey and the CHA need to take more of a leadership role on some of the issues I've discussed in this chapter. For example, while they do a great job of keeping up with changes in rules and organizing coaching programs, I feel they should be more forthright in setting out limits on the number of games kids play in a season, and even the length of that season. Further, I think serious attention needs to be paid to ways of improving practices and ensuring that fun and skills are given priority over competition and winning. The video *Fun and Games on Ice* is a great place to start exploring the possibilities for yourself (see Appendix 5).

What can you do? Particularly as a new hockey parent, you may feel your role is to keep quiet and watch. I disagree. Get involved. You can assist on the bench, or take a coaching course. Attend your local association's meetings. You don't have to contribute right away, but by getting involved you'll soon become conversant in the issues that shape children's hockey and you'll be in a better position to convey your ideas to your local association. Also, if you want to find out more about the organizational structure of your local association and USA Hockey or the CHA, give them a call or write to request whatever information they have available (they both have websites, too).

At minimum, I urge you not to be afraid to ask questions—whether it's about too many games or the qualifications and general approach of your son's or daughter's coach. Even if the local association is reluctant to change, pressure from parents for more practice time and fewer games—for fundamentals and fun—will eventually have an effect.

Hockey is enormous fun. It's even better when it's taught the right way.

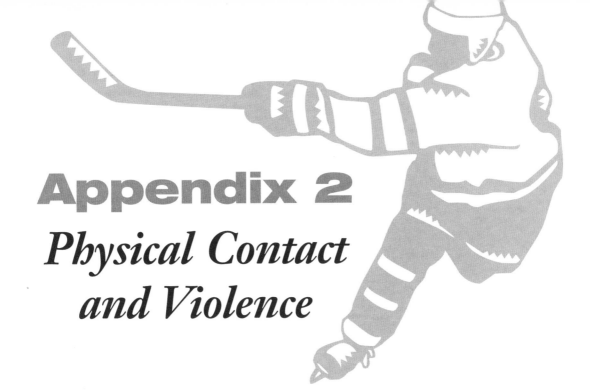

Appendix 2
Physical Contact and Violence

Hockey has gained a nasty reputation for violence over the years and this is largely due to the professional ranks. Kids' hockey remains a safe, fun and exciting sport. It's natural, of course, to be worried. In this appendix I go over the different aspects of body contact in hockey—from the unavoidable (which is part of the game) to the intolerable.

CHECKING AND BODY CONTACT

As I discussed in Chapter 3, checking just means trying to get the puck away from another player or covering an opponent. It's a central part of the game. Body-checking—using the body to force an opponent off the puck—isn't allowed in kids' hockey for the most part. But it's perfectly legal for a player to use his or her stick to lift an opponent's stick or bat the puck away. When checking gets too rough, penalties are called. See Chapter 2 for a list of rules and penalties.

Many first-time hockey parents are worried about injuries caused by body-checking. And if all you know about hockey is the pro brand, glimpsed on TV, you might agree. Those guys hit hard, and it's rare for a player to escape injury for an entire career. Do I think this a reason to steer your child away from hockey? My

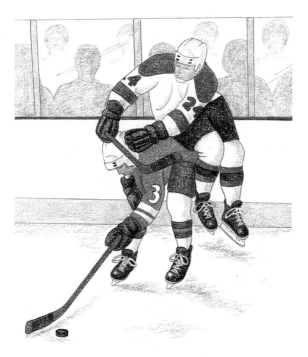

The Big League Body-check

Professional players can dish out hard hits like this one, but they know how to give and take a body-check.

answer is no. Barring some very unusual combination of circumstances, your child is not going to be involved in full-contact hockey for several years, if at all.

Most hockey associations do not allow body-checking (as opposed to body contact) before the players are 12. Girls' and women's hockey associations never allow it, and some mixed or boys' house leagues may ban it in all age groups. For the most part, rep (all-star) hockey is the only program that permits body-checking. The simplest way to avoid body-checking completely is to keep your child out of rep and select hockey.

But body contact in hockey isn't avoidable. It's a fast-paced game played in a rink with boards four feet high. At minimum, players are going to run into each other as they scramble for the puck. For this reason, children's equipment needs to be of good quality and properly fitted even when no body-checking is allowed. For me, injuries caused by accidental collisions are more of a concern than the imagined dangers of body-checking. I talk about safety and playing smart more fully in Chapter 3.

BODY-CHECKING: THE DEBATE

The Canadian Academy of Sports Medicine (CASM), of which I am a member, has recommended that body-checking be eliminated at all playing levels that are not designed as training grounds for professional hockey. The academy also questioned whether body-checking should even begin at 12, because serious injuries begin to appear in Peewee hockey (ages 12 and 13.) A Canadian study that compared checking and non-checking leagues at the Peewee level players showed that 88 percent of fractures were related to body-checking and that fractures were 12 times more frequent in players and leagues that allowed body-checking.

It's also true that not all 12-year-olds, say, are equal. One may be nearly full-grown while the other is still a small child. The difference can be as much as five years in what I call physiological age—age as measured by size and strength. Organized hockey groups kids according to age, and we sometimes find small 12-year-olds being checked by huge ones. The American Academy of Pediatrics has recommended grouping players by weight, size, physical condition, maturation and skill instead of by age alone. Most other contact sports—football and wrestling, for example—do so. Some girls' hockey leagues follow this practice as well.

Medical science has shown that growth plates in bones are more susceptible to injury during the growth spurts of puberty. Consequently, the CASM has urged that body-checking should not begin until Midget (16 to 17 years old), when there is less of a size difference and growth spurts are mostly over. In a position statement in 1988, the CASM also suggested that limited body-checking could be introduced at the Bantam level (14 to 15 years).

On the other hand, some experts, such as Dr. Tom Pashby, think that rep or all-star players should be taught body-checking techniques from the day they begin elite hockey. Pashby is a world-famous eye surgeon, who played a key role in introducing full facial protection, which dramatically reduced serious eye and facial injuries in minor hockey. His argument is that waiting until age 14 or 16 to introduce body-checking would be hazardous to elite players, who need to be taught proper checking techniques from a young age. By the time they reach Midget age, elite players are at high risk for spinal cord injuries because of their size and speed. Pashby thinks they'd be better off learning how to give and take a body-check earlier, when they're smaller and slower and the risks of injury are consequently lower.

Certainly, Pashby makes a good argument. I see younger players going into the boards and corners, heads down, with no regard for safety because they know they cannot get hit. Perhaps if they were in danger of a body-check, they'd be more alert. More to the point, perhaps they wouldn't arrive at the Peewee level with bad, dangerous habits.

However, as a hockey coach of many years and as a sports doctor, I'm not completely convinced by either side of the body-checking debate. Personally, I'd allow body-checking at the Peewee level, but only in the neutral zone (between the blue lines.) Then I'd allow full ice body-checking at Bantam. Sooner or later, if a player is talented and wants to aim for a professional career, body-checking is going to happen. I believe phasing it in could make the transition easier and safer.

As well, most of the dangerous situations occur in the end zones, when a player is trying to dig out a puck against the boards; checks in the neutral zone, by contrast, tend to occur while a player is carrying the puck in open ice, so they are less dangerous. If body-checking started only at the Peewee level, and if the first year or two of body-checking were limited, I think it would be safer.

But I also think we *must* educate kids from the beginning about being safe on the ice. That way they won't form the bad habits that can lead to later injury.

My beliefs on this issue are reflected in my hockey school teaching and my coaching. As I explained in Chapter 3, I encourage young players always to be aware of where they are on the ice (particularly if they're within a stride or two of the boards) and of other players near them (opponents *and* teammates). Near the boards is the real danger zone on the ice. Falling or getting knocked down away from the boards isn't a real problem, although it might hurt for a minute or two. But even a simple fall or awkward stumble in the danger zone can cause trouble.

Coaching or teaching, I always remind my players of the following tips. You might do the same every now and then for your child.

- Play with the head up at all times.

- Play with the stick down.

- Know where opposing players are.

- Never go straight into the boards. Always go in at an angle (see diagram on page 58).

- In a puck scramble, play against the boards, not a few feet out.

- Play with the skates in line with the boards.

A player with the head down and the skates at right angles (or close to it) near the boards is in a dangerous position. Whether body-checking is allowed or not, the player could get knocked right into the boards—an open invitation to a spinal injury. Fortunately, as a coach I haven't seen an injury like this, but I've heard about them. Kids must be taught to play smart. Tell your child (and any other player who'll listen to you): Do not put yourself in a position where you can be hit from behind, even accidentally, and driven into the boards head-first. The child could also get driven into the butt end of the stick when it hits the boards just before he or she does.

I teach contact confidence at my hockey school. I have the kids go through some drills that get them used to body-checking and contact at a young age (see Chapter 3). But at the same time they never stop hearing from me to keep their heads up and their sticks down. Not all hockey schools do this, but I think they should. The rep team I coach for has limited body-checking; but even for house league, contact confidence goes a long way to getting kids to play smarter on the ice, and it also helps get them ready if they make the step up to rep (or even if they keep playing house league as they get older). This has become more important over the past decades as improved equipment (especially full face shields) has left many young players feeling invincible on the ice. Players need to be aware that there are still dangers on the ice— from nasty stick-work to getting hit from behind. By teaching them to respect each other and to play smart, we can help kids avoid injury on the ice.

FIGHTING

If all you know about hockey comes from watching the occasional NHL game on television, you might think that fighting is an integral part of the game. It's a forgivable mistake, but it's dead wrong—especially in kids' hockey. Dropping the gloves and taking a sock at the other player is not tolerated in any league for children. The penalty for fighting is usually an automatic game suspension. In some cases, the punishment may be more severe.

So don't hesitate to enroll your child in hockey if it's the idea of fighting that turns you off. It is, by and large, a nonissue. In fact, unless they're egged on, most kids don't even think of starting a fight on the ice.

The National Hockey League is another story. As long as there has been an NHL, there has been fighting—and discussion, debate and controversy over fighting. The league has tried to tone down the fighting, with some success. An antibrawling rule has eliminated the bench-clearing scrums that used to occur. And the rule that gives an extra penalty to the player who deliberately instigates a fight is a good start. But perhaps because violence sells, the NHL has not banned fighting altogether. So there are still good players being turned into fight-on-command goons by professional organizations (look what happened to Nick Kypreos, who was a prolific goal-scorer in Junior). I wonder how many parents (not the readers of this book, of course) are keeping their child out of the sport because of fighting in the NHL. I also wonder how many fans have abandoned hockey because of fighting.

The NHL would like to ignore the fighting issue despite the moral conundrum in which it often puts parents. Professional players are many of our children's role models. How do we—either as parents or coaches—explain to 9-year-olds that fighting has no part in hockey when their heroes are battling it out on television? Luckily for those of us who love the game for its speed and grace, most kids still idolize skilled players like Mats Sundin and Wayne Gretzky, rather than scrappers like Marty McSorley or Stu (the Grim Reaper) Grimson.

You have to explain to your child that the NHL players are making a living playing the game and that hockey at this level is entertainment much like a staged wrestling act, although the fights are real. Don't ignore fighting in the professional and junior ranks. Instead, emphasize that *you* don't think it is acceptable behavior. Praise the skilled hockey players, who are scoring goals and making nice plays. Also encourage your kids, when they're old enough, to emulate players who know how to throw a legal body check, not those who trip, hold and elbow.

Having said all that, how do we teach an aspiring hockey player that fighting is not right? First, it must be made clear that we live in a society that doesn't tolerate violence. It's never the right way to solve a conflict. We don't tolerate it at home or school, on the field or rink. Explain to your child what would happen if you, the parent, resorted to violence every time you had a conflict at work.

There's a rule on my hockey team that a player stays off for a shift, even after the penalty is over, if he or she takes a stupid penalty. Kids need to learn sooner rather than later that cross-checking or elbowing or letting loose with a punch is wrong and has negative consequences. If the referee didn't see a serious infraction, that player's coach, in my view, is responsible for instilling a lesson in that player. On one occasion, I kept a player on the bench for a whole game after he'd whacked an opponent with his stick. I told the parents what I'd seen the boy do and they agreed that it was important that the child be taught a lesson.

Most fights happen in front of the net, after a whistle. The players have been battling for the puck, and many times a forward gets what seems like a cheap shot from the defense player. There's no question that it can be tough for players to keep their tempers in check when they feel they've taken a cheap shot. But most of the time these jabs don't hurt, and often the referee will call a penalty against the other guy. By retaliating, the player only costs his or her team a power play advantage. Tell your child the best response is to skate away and then score a goal next shift. Beat them on the scoreboard, not in the alley.

But what if your child does get in a fight? In the early years, it's unlikely, of course. But what if? In the first place, two 7-year-olds flailing away are unlikely to cause any damage, especially when you consider that they're wearing full equipment, including a facemask. After all, even a scrap in the playground at that age rarely causes anything more than hurt feelings. Secondly, the ref will break it up pretty quickly. In the NHL, they tend to let the scuffle go on until someone falls to the ice, but in kids' hockey, the officials will get involved immediately.

So, there's almost no physical danger. But as a parent and as a hockey coach, I'd want the ref to throw both players out of the game. If they are not ejected—sometimes the referee feels the scuffle wasn't a "real" fight and hands out two-minute penalties—then I would hope the coaches would sit them out the rest of the game. How else can a child learn that fighting is not tolerated?

Even more important than sitting a player on the bench is for the parent to sit down with the player and find out what happened. And why. Hear the child out. Try to understand his or her point of view. Above all, don't make light of the issue. You are the key to your child's understanding of the game.

One other point: There are bullies everywhere, even in kids' hockey leagues. Sometimes they're parents, sometimes they're coaches and sometimes they're players. If another player starts taking punches at your kid, he or she has the right to self-defense, just as if it were happening in the playground or on the street. Self-defense is an important concept; fighting is wrong, but being a punching bag isn't any better.

With any kind of luck, the refs and the coaches will recognize what happened and deal with the bully appropriately.

At the same time you as a parent must control your emotions—something that can be hard to do when your child is in trouble. Above all, *don't* make a scene in the stands by screaming at or—worse yet—attacking the other players' parents or coaches. I have seen this happen. It's ugly.

Fighting is, unfortunately, still part of the professional game. But it's not part of children's hockey and should not be something for you to worry about when your child wants to play. Hockey is a game of speed, grace and beauty—not fighting and brutality.

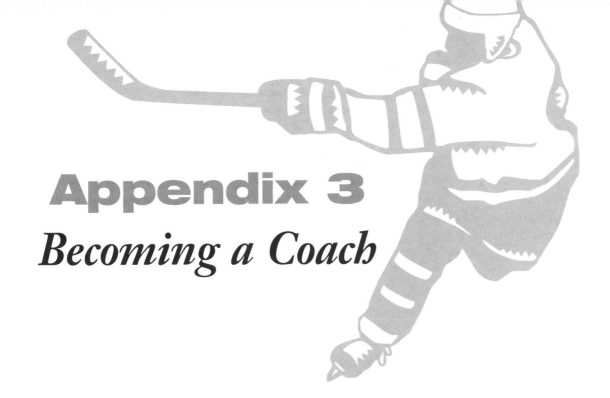

Appendix 3
Becoming a Coach

Coaching kids is a lot of fun. Hockey associations are always looking for volunteer coaches and if you're interested, there are lots of courses you can take to prepare for this challenging position. Make no mistake, however, good coaching takes a great deal of time and energy. And like most things in life, the more you put into it the more you get out of it. But if you enjoy hockey, coaching can be great fun and you'll learn a lot about yourself in the process. Although I taught myself much about hockey drills and conditioning by reading almost everything available on the subject, when I decided I wanted to get involved in coaching rep (all-star) hockey, I had to take the coaching certification course. And it's a good thing I did. On this two-day weekend course I learned some new tricks and met some of the most committed individuals involved in amateur hockey. In this appendix, after discussing assistant coaches and trainers, I offer some thoughts on the role of the coach. I also touch on the issue of coaching one's own child because this seems to be a problem at times. Lastly, I address how one can actually get started in coaching and what courses are available (first in Canada and then the United States).

ASSISTANT COACHES AND TRAINERS

I've often been asked by people at the rink if you need to know how to skate to be a coach. The short answer is yes. All the good will in the world won't make up for a certain level of skills that a coach needs to know. A coach can get away with not being a good skater behind the bench at a game, but at practice the coach has to be out on the ice running the practice, putting the kids through drills, and teaching skills. That's the job. In my experience most coaches have played the game as kids (and some continue in adult amateur leagues) and have mastered many of the basic skills I talked about in Chapter 3. In coaching courses these individuals learn how to better teach these skills to kids. However, the basic skills themselves can't really be learned in a weekend course. In truth, it takes years of experience to become a good teacher. If you can't skate very well or haven't mastered most of the basic skills, you might be better off helping out as a trainer or assistant coach. As assistant coach you'll be the coach's right hand in managing the potential chaos of a children's hockey practice. As trainer you'll also help with practices and behind the bench at games and be in charge of any injuries (you'll need first-aid certification). If you end up under the wing of a good and experienced coach you'll learn a lot. After a season or two of skating with the kids during practices and standing behind the bench at games, you can decide if you're ready to move into a coaching position. Either way, good volunteers are always welcome—especially in house league where finding enough adults to properly staff a team can be a challenge.

THE ROLE OF THE COACH

The most important role for a coach in any kids' sport is to keep it fun and challenging. If the kids aren't having fun then they will be impossible to teach. But fun is only part of the equation. As a coach you are a tremendous role model for your players. There are lots of excellent studies available that show that to a child the coach is one of the most important role models they have growing up. So, in being a coach you bear a good deal of responsibility. Not only do you need to successfully impart hockey skills to the children, you need to be a model of fairness and levelheadedness. Whether dealing with your young players, their parents, the other adults helping to run the team or the opposing team's staff in a game, you are, like it or not, a model for those kids of how to interact with all sorts of individuals. Getting angry and yelling at the ref or the other team's coach is a good way to instill a lack of respect in the players for yourself. So, be respectful to the kids, the referees and the opposing teams. Be cheerful and encouraging rather than aggressive and critical—the kids and the team as a whole will benefit if you seem happy being around them and coaching the team for them. Dress neatly, take care of the team's equipment and show up on time.

And that's not all. As a good coach you should try to educate yourself in the areas of skill development and coaching techniques. All sorts of books and videos should be available through your local association or library. If you're not prepared to put some effort into it, there is almost no point in becoming involved. Make it your hobby. It sure beats sitting in front of the television (well, except for hockey).

At the purely practical level, perhaps the most important element a coach needs to get a handle on is developing an effective practice. But let me ask you to remember that no matter how seriously you or the other team staff take the job of coaching, the kids are there to have fun. So developing an effective practice that involves all the kids and maintains an element of fun sounds much easier than it is. This is where your research in the library looking at different books and videos comes in. Once you've established a basic set of drills and routines for the kids (remember, you can do some drills at one practice and others at next week's), prepare to be flexible with them. You can also try inventing some new drills of your own. But keep things flowing in your practice—which is another way of saying don't let your idea of the perfect drill get in the way of the kids having fun and learning at the same time. They're just kids, right? Sometimes just a little inventiveness and flexibility can turn a boring drill from a book into a rollicking exercise for the kids. Just because something has been done one way in the past doesn't mean it's the right way for your team and its chemistry. I think that almost anyone can stand at center ice, blow the whistle and have the kids skate up and down the ice. But as a role model and educator (which is what a coach is) you need to teach the game of hockey, and teach it in a fun and creative way. So don't hesitate to let the kids play some games in practice from time to time. Three-on-three with quick shifts is fun, or have them go five-on-five and put the goalies in too. In my view, a lot of skills are being learned in the apparent mayhem of a Mini-Mite or Tyke game.

And don't forget about your goaltender. He or she really makes up about 20 percent of your team during a game since this player never leaves the ice. So being a good coach also means learning about goaltending and trying to teach this player some skills. Which isn't easy. If you're having trouble helping your goaltender, don't be afraid to ask for some help from your association, or another coach, or invite a local Junior goaltender out to a practice.

Overall, if you are the right person for the job, coaching is a great experience. But it is not easy. It simply isn't enough to have played the game as a kid or adolescent and then expect to go out on the ice and teach kids the game of hockey. It requires some work and preparation. And whether you are coaching house league or rep, you still need to put 100 percent effort into being a coach. A house-league player needs to learn to stop just as much as a rep player. At the end of the day, teaching basic skills is the cornerstone of coaching. The respect and affection you earn by being responsible, fair, flexible and decent is what allows the teaching of those skills to effectively take place.

COACHING YOUR OWN CHILD

In most instances coaches of children's hockey will have a child of their own on the team. Why? Well, if you have children, it's fairly difficult to justify the time spent coaching someone else's kids rather than your own. That said, I think that coaching your own child can be a very positive experience for both you and your child. But if you have more than one child in the sport, then you'll have to try and rotate whose team you're involved with from year to year. As coach of your own child, you tend to be a little harder on him or her. It's important to be aware of this and a good check is to ask yourself if you'd be censuring or pushing a child as hard if he or she weren't your own. If the answer is no, then backing off might be a good idea. It's important for the game to remain fun for your child too. Think back, when you were a child did you enjoy your leisure activities when you had a parent standing over you the whole time telling you what to do, and worse, what you were doing wrong?

When a game or practice is over, don't bring it home—not the bad stuff anyway. Leave it at the rink and in the dressing room. Remember, your child is expecting you to act as a parent and not just as a coach. Encourage rather than criticize. Ask if he or she likes the practices and what drills you could do next time for everyone. Your child can be a good gauge of how the other players are finding the practices and games. And don't forget to ask your child if he or she is really enjoying hockey. Just because you're putting in all that effort doesn't mean it's the best sport or arrangement for your child.

As for other parents, if you don't know it already, you'll soon learn that they will be watching you very closely as you carry out your responsibilities as coach. Believe me, they will make sure your child doesn't get any more ice time than theirs. The bottom line is you have to be fair to all the kids—you'll need a clear conscience when an angry parent starts challenging some of your coaching decisions. If a discipline problem arises with your child on the ice—in practice or at a game—a good idea is to have someone else address the problem (the assistant coach or the trainer). This way your child doesn't get the impression you're picking on him or her. On my son's team, the team staff got together before the season started and we decided that each of us would address any behavior problems that arose with each other's children but not our own. This way we avoided giving the impression to our own kids that we were picking on them.

I've really enjoyed coaching my two older boys and I look forward to coaching my youngest because I can honestly say that it's a positive experience for me, and my children really enjoy having me as part of their team.

COACHING CERTIFICATIONS

In Canada, coaching in house league doesn't always require certification—depending on the local association. However, if you want to coach select or rep (all-star), then a coaching certificate will be required. In the United States coaching at any level requires appropriate certification. Typically, individuals wanting to coach a rep or select team will have to apply to the local association where a selection committee will decide among all the applicants. Here's where higher coaching certification levels can be a real help. However, selection committees (especially in Canada) don't necessarily give priority to certification levels over years of playing and coaching experience. All coaching certifications charge a fee for the courses (it varies from association to association)—the fee covers the qualified instructors hired by the local association, ice rental, manuals and audio-visual materials. By the way, except for CHIP (see below), all coaching certifications in Canada and the United States require periodic refresher courses to maintain status.

THE CANADIAN HOCKEY INITIATION PROGRAM (CHIP)

The basic minimum for coaching certification in Canada is a program called the Canadian Hockey Initiation Program (CHIP). The one-day course is offered through your local association and is designed to provide new coaches with enough information on basic hockey skills to allow them to instruct youngsters between the ages of 5 and 9. The coach is equipped with a manual that specifically shows him or her how to teach certain skills to kids. Many organizations require the basic CHIP certification to step behind the bench as a coach in house league; others may require the more thorough National Coaching Certificate (see below). Even if your local association doesn't insist on it at the house-league level, I strongly urge you to take at least the CHIP course and the first level of the National Coaching Certificate Program.

THE NATIONAL COACHING CERTIFICATE PROGRAM (CANADA)

In 1972 the Canadian Hockey Association, which governs amateur hockey across Canada, began its first formal coaching clinics called the National Coaching Certificate Program (NCCP). Then, as now, the objective of the NCCP is to enhance the quality of coaching throughout Canada to ensure that young players receive the best possible instruction and training (this organization, by the way, has been imitated throughout the world). There are four certification levels available through the NCCP. For rep or select teams coaches must have at least level I. The advanced levels may become more interesting to you as you gain more experience. If you decide to climb up the coaching ladder to more competitive teams and higher age brackets, the more advanced coaching certifications may be required by your local association.

The first level, Level I, is simply called coach level. Certification requires a two-day course where participants learn the general role of a coach, how to communicate with players, how to organize a practice, how to teach basic skills and how to keep the game fun for the kids. As part of the course you'll be required to go on the ice for approximately two hours.

Level II, or intermediate as it's often referred to, is designed for the coach working at a more competitive level (rep or all-star) and who wishes to enhance his or her knowledge and skills. The three-day (21-hour) course examines the coaching process in greater depth. Issues around the physical development and mental growth of young athletes are given some attention and there is a section on the recognition and management of injuries. Team tactics (rather than exclusively individual skills) are given special attention and there is also a section on goaltending. You'll spend about four hours on the ice for this course.

In Level III, or Advanced Level I, coaches with several years' experience at competitive levels learn complicated team systems, off-ice conditioning, nutrition, motivating players and player psychology (on and off the ice). Participants are also taught how to produce and interpret team and player statistics. This is a 30-hour course held over several days and takes place once each year in every province. Interested coaches apply to the NCCP and are selected by a committee that will contact the local association to solicit review of the applicant's prior performance and competence.

The fourth level is called Advanced Level II and is for the really serious coach with at least five years of coaching experience. The 65-hour course is held every two years in Canada with candidates being selected from across the country by the Canadian Hockey Association. Part of the program is coordinated with the Coaching

Association of Canada (which represents coaches from nearly all sports). Coaches learn more advanced skills and also spend time on the psychology and physical conditioning of advanced hockey players (university, Junior and professional).

USA HOCKEY'S COACHING ACHIEVEMENT PROGRAM

USA Hockey has developed a coaching education system consisting of a volunteer track and a career track. With the volunteer track the coach can progress through four levels—similar to the Canadian NCCP program on which it is modelled. The four levels are called Course level, Associate level, Intermediate level and Advanced level. As a coach progresses through the levels, it allows him or her to coach higher caliber hockey. With the Course level, coaches can head house-league teams up to the age of Atom and rep Mite teams. The Associate level allows for the coaching of teams up to the age of Midget house league and Squirt rep teams. The Intermediate level allows for the coaching of Midget house league and up to the level of Bantam rep. The Advanced level permits coaching at all levels of amateur hockey up to Junior A excluding college teams. This progressive system is somewhat different from its Canadian counterpart in that in Canada higher coaching certification is not always obligatory for more advanced hockey. However, the concepts and skills taught by both programs are basically the same, as are the time requirements. Signing up for courses is usually done through the local or district association.

The career track in coaching certification is for individuals who coach (or hope to) for a living; this includes college, Junior and professional coaches. After taking the four volunteer level courses, career coaches can continue with Master, Elite and High Performance levels. These individuals spend much more time learning team tactics, psychology, training (off- and on-ice), nutrition and high-performance skills.

Another organization, the American Sports Education Program (formerly known as the American Coaching Effectiveness Program), offers a great deal of excellent material to the coach or parent. This program has put out a great book called *Coaching Youth Hockey*. It gives a solid overview of what it takes to be a hockey coach. ASEP also provides information on first aid and nutrition for all athletes. I encourage you to contact them (they're listed in Appendix 5).

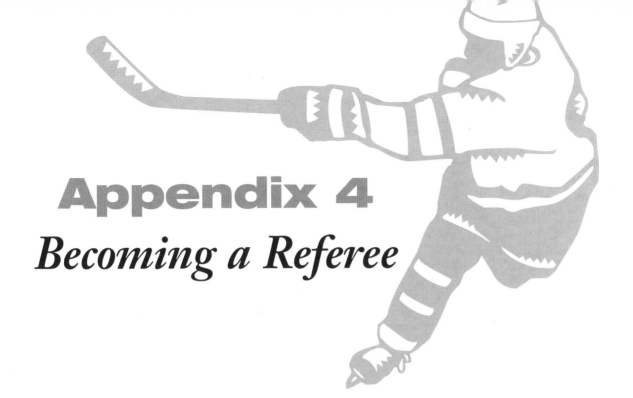

Appendix 4
Becoming a Referee

Maybe a more appropriate title for this chapter is "Why Become a Referee?" Who in their right mind would want to be subjected to such abuse? Well, let me reassure you it is not all bad. In fact, as hard as it may be to believe, referees are paid by local minor hockey associations. So if you want to find out how you can have fun skating and get paid at the same time, read on. It is a great part-time job for teens and an excellent way to keep fit for an adult.

In its early years organized hockey was officiated with only one referee, and for the first nine years of its existence the NHL used only one official in games. Those first lone referees rang a bell to signal a stoppage in play and sometime later the whistle was introduced. And there was no formal referee school—former players usually refereed the games and called them as they saw fit. In 1941, the NHL introduced the one referee (wearing red armbands) and two linesmen system. In today's modern NHL game we now have two referees and two linesmen.

As for myself I refereed for close to 10 years in the Ontario Minor Hockey Association. Eventually I worked my way up to a full Level 3 referee (I will explain the levels in a minute). I love to skate, so for me refereeing was a great way to earn a few dollars and enjoy myself at the same time—refs and goalies stay on the ice for the entire game.

I've heard it said that refereeing a hockey game is probably the most challenging job in team sports. And as a referee, there is no question that you take a lot of abuse.

You certainly have to develop a tough outer shell. But sometimes that isn't enough. Recently the abuse seems to be getting more out of hand and this has caused many fine referees to leave the game. It has also led to ref shortages in many associations. Occasionally verbal abuse has spilled over into the physical. Fortunately this is not a common scenario; the few incidents have been at advanced levels of hockey. As for the verbal abuse, kids' hockey is nothing like Junior or the NHL. Remember, the NHL is a business and it's there to entertain us. The referees are part of the package. The abuse the officials take on TV is not tolerated in youth hockey. If players or coaches swear at the referee, then they are ejected from the game.

However, I sometimes think referees often bring such problems on themselves. I firmly believe that if a referee does a good job and understands the rule book completely, he or she will run into little trouble on the ice. A referee must not let a game get out of hand. He or she must recognize if this is happening and take prompt action. From my observations of many of today's referees at the local level, they appear to be lacking enough training and knowledge of the game to do this. (Some aren't really good enough skaters to keep up with the play, which means they miss penalties and off-sides.) Knowing the rule book inside-out is one of the two best ways to avoid ambiguity and to instill respect in fans and players. The other way is to be firm and confident in the decisions one makes on the ice. If confidence or knowledge is lacking, a referee will always be vulnerable to the verbal slights thrown his or her way. Being fair goes without saying.

In children's hockey, most games are officiated by two referees with equal power. As the children get older and the games get faster, most leagues adopt the system of two linesmen and one referee. As in all levels of hockey, the referee is basically responsible for signaling goals and calling penalties. The linesmen drop the majority of face-offs and call off-sides and icings.

REFEREE CERTIFICATION

If you're still serious about becoming a referee, then let's get down to the meat and potatoes of how it's done. Referee certification clinics are not free in Canada so expect a reasonable fee that covers the costs of management to coordinate the program, the trainers and ice time. Sometimes your local hockey association will contribute part of the cost. One way of finding out about upcoming referee certification clinics is through your association's referee-in-chief. Most associations will have a referee-in-chief who is familiar with the scheduling and staffing of the clinics and who conducts the evaluations of candidates. This individual is also responsible for scheduling referees for all of the association's games. By the way, the amount a referee is paid for each game typically depends on the referee's level of experience, the age level of the teams and caliber of play (house league or rep). In play-off games for the rep (or all-star) level, referees are often brought in from a neutral town or city to prevent any biases toward the home team. For regular season play at the rep level, it is the home team's local association that typically provides the referees.

Once you have become a referee, whether in the United States or Canada, periodic recertification and refresher courses are necessary to maintain your level.

CANADIAN HOCKEY OFFICIATING PROGRAM (CHOP)

In Canada, minor hockey referees are certified and governed by an organization called the Canadian Hockey Officiating Program. CHOP operates under the Canadian Hockey Association and is the nationally recognized development program for all on-ice officials. The program is structured into six levels of certification. Programs are held every year, usually in early autumn before the beginning of the hockey season, and most often are organized by the local hockey associations. In most cases, you can find out where and when the next clinic is offered by contacting your local hockey association. As I mentioned earlier, the clinics are not free so find out ahead of time how much your local association is charging for the course.

Let's take a closer look at the six CHOP levels.

Level 1 is an introductory beginners' course to prepare new or young officials to referee children's house-league hockey. The clinic is usually a day-long course with some on-ice participation. There is a written exam at the end of the course on which a score of at least 70 percent is required for certification.

Level 2 is an extension of Level 1 with the proviso that candidates must be 16 years of age or older. It is also a day-long clinic and again you must obtain a minimum of 70 percent on a written national exam. With a Level 2 certification, you may referee at the rep (or all-star) level of children's hockey.

Level 3 is a more in-depth course that prepares officials to referee minor hockey play-offs and also act as linesmen at higher categories. To qualify for Level 3 you must have a Level 2 certification and have refereed a minimum of one year at that level. You must obtain 80 percent on a written national exam and then pass a practical on-ice evaluation conducted by a qualified CHOP supervisor. The on-ice evaluation can be very stressful (much like a driver's examination). The CHOP supervisor is on the lookout for every little mistake. Out of all the exams I have been through, including medical school, for some reason this experience stands out as a particularly stressful event. You may come across the occasional referee with Level 3 certification in minor hockey. These refs are exceptional skaters and really serious about their job.

Level 4 prepares officials to referee up to the Senior (19 years plus) or Junior (16 to 20) level or to act as linesmen for major Junior A hockey. Participants in this program must be invited by their branch, must have a Level 3 certification and have refereed for a minimum of one year at this level. The course is held over two days and the candidate must obtain a minimum of 80 percent on the written national exam and pass a practical on-ice evaluation.

Level 5 officials are qualified to referee major Junior hockey and at the university level. This is an intense course and candidates must obtain 90 percent on a written exam and pass a practical on-ice evaluation along with a fitness and skating test.

Level 6 is the top official level. These officials are permitted to officiate at National Championships and World Championships. Level 6 is an intense four-day instructional clinic.

USA HOCKEY OFFICIATING PROGRAM

In the United States, officials are trained through the USA Hockey Officiating Program. USA Hockey will register candidates (male or female) between the age of 11 and 70. The goal of the program is to provide opportunities for officials to gain the proper experience at the lower levels of competition and to promote the more experienced and talented officials to the higher ranks of officiating. The programs are usually conducted in the fall just before the new hockey season. All seminars are conducted free of charge. The program is divided into levels of achievement. First-year officials register as Level 1 officials. However, if you have prior experience, then your case may be reviewed by the referee-in-chief to place you at a higher level.

Level 1 officials may officiate games at age levels of 8 to 12 years. Certification is obtained by writing an open-book examination on the rules of hockey.

Level 2 candidates have one to two years' experience and learn more advanced techniques of officiating at a hockey seminar spread over several days. Again, there's an open-book exam. Level 2 referees may officiate for all divisions under the age of 14.

Level 3 officials are qualified to referee any games played by teams in the 17 or under age classification. Candidates enroll in a seminar that takes place over several days and finish up by writing an exam. These officials may also act as linesmen for Junior hockey.

Level 4 officials are the highest qualified officials under USA Hockey. Level 4 allows officials to referee Junior, high-school and higher level games. To qualify, the referee must have two years' experience at Level 3. There is a written as well as an on-ice skating exam as part of the qualifying process.

As members of USA Hockey officiating, referees are protected with liability insurance along with medical and dental coverage. They are also provided with updated rule books and a newsletter called *Stripes Newsletter* issued four times per year. To find out about a clinic in your area, contact the local supervisor of officials or the district referee-in-chief for your local association. These names are easily obtainable through USA Hockey. USA Hockey also conducts various camps for elite officials and programs to train referee instructors.

EQUIPMENT FOR REFEREES

Like anyone else on the ice, referees wear specialized equipment. They must wear a certified hockey helmet and most associations insist that refs wear a half visor to protect the eyes. Traditionally the referee's helmet is black. Since there is no type of specialized referee helmet available, refs wear one of the types that players use. Make sure the helmet fits correctly and replace it if the lining becomes cracked or the shell damaged. It is just as important for a referee to have a good-quality helmet as any other player.

Refs also need to wear a protective cup (a jock or jill). Genital injuries can be very painful; remember that at every face-off an official is at risk from a blow of a player's stick. And a wayward slap shot is a real danger. Again there are no special types of protective cups for officials.

Specialized pants that hug the waist and upper leg much like a girdle are available for referees. The padding is thinner than that used in regular hockey pants, which means the padded girdle can be worn under the black pants traditionally worn by referees. Specialized referee pants are available at sporting goods stores; however, polyester-style dress pants with ample room for movement will also suffice.

All referees should also wear elbow pads. The elbow pads made specifically for referees are usually lighter weight and allow greater freedom of movement; however, regular hockey elbow pads will do. The elbow is an important area to be protected at all times since it isn't uncommon for a referee to fall and land on the hand and elbow region.

The last piece of protective equipment for referees are shin pads. Again there are specialized pads available for referees. These are lighter weight and less bulky than a player's pads. The shin pads protect from any stray pucks and sticks, particularly around face-offs.

Finally, the most important piece of equipment is the black-and-white striped referee shirt. There is an old saying in hockey which goes, "black and white and never right," but don't let this get you down. Make sure you iron your referee shirt on a regular basis. Part of the job is looking professional at all times. Remember, you have to gain and maintain the respect of the coaches, players and fans.

Oh yes, I almost forgot, the whistle. Do not buy a cheap one. The cheaper models tend to freeze up under cold conditions. Remember to keep a spare in the locker room.

If you want to get really fancy, you can buy a specialized equipment bag for lugging your referee gear from game to game. These are very handy since they usually have a separate compartment for stowing a neatly folded sweater.

SUMMING UP

As an official, I feel one of the referee's major roles is prevention of injury. So it's not a bad idea to have some type of first-aid certification to help out the coaching staff if a player is injured. Also, referees should inspect the ice surface before the game for debris or cracks to prevent players from falling and possibly hurting themselves. And once on the ice, the referee should lead by example, which means wearing properly maintained equipment at all games. Further, it's important to enforce the rules that prevent major injuries, such as checking from behind, boarding and spearing. Regardless of the score or situation, always call the game by the rule book; playing favorites is all too apparent from the stands or the bench. Remember, as a referee it's important to educate coaches and players about the rules and why they exist—this will give them a better understanding of injury prevention and, yes, simple fairness.

Appendix 5
Organizations and Resources for Amateur Hockey

Your local hockey association is probably all you need to be familiar with during your child's first year or two of hockey. But you should be aware that local hockey associations are the all-important base of a pyramid of organizations that culminates (in the United States) in USA Hockey and (in Canada) in the Canadian Hockey Association. These organizations are the governing bodies for amateur hockey. In the last analysis, they provide the structure that lets your child, and hundreds of thousands of others, have a safe, fun time at the rink. The CHA, for instance, had well over 500,000 players registered in 1999–2000. All told, more than 4 million Canadians are involved as players, coaches, officials and volunteers. And that doesn't include parents. The numbers for the USA Hockey association aren't far behind—around 400,000 players in 1999–2000 and about another 100,000 coaches and officials. USA Hockey doesn't estimate the number of volunteers.

Both organizations promote safety, offer extensive programs to develop coaches and referees, and work to keep hockey fair and fun for all.

USA Hockey
1775 Bob Johnson Dr.
Colorado Springs, CO
8096-4090
(719) 576-8724
(719) 538-1160 (fax)

Canadian Hockey Association
1600 Prom. James Naismith Dr.
Suite 607
Gloucester, ON
K1B 5N4
(613) 748-5613
(613) 748-5709 (fax)

THE HOCKEY DEVELOPMENT CENTRE AND WOMEN'S HOCKEY

One of the best resources for amateur hockey, whether you live in the United States or Canada, is the Hockey Development Centre for Ontario. This organization was established in 1984 to promote safety, education and development of amateur hockey in Ontario. The HDCO is also an important resource for parents, coaches and hockey organizers. It has a host of videos, manuals, drill books, coaching aids, information for team trainers and resources for referees to improve their skills. It also publishes a newspaper called *Ice Times*, which is usually available for free at many hockey arenas.

Hockey Development Centre for Ontario
1185 Eglinton Ave. E.
Suite 301
Toronto, ON
M3C 3C6
(416) 426-7252
(416) 426-7348 (fax)

Again, whether you live in the United States or Canada, the Ontario Women's Hockey Association is one of the best resources for information on women's and girls' hockey in all of North America. It was established in 1975 and is one of the oldest organizations of its kind. The OWHA was instrumental in bringing women's hockey to the world stage, including the Olympics. The association has information on equipment and women's tournaments, and even about setting up a girls' hockey association in your community.

Ontario Women's Hockey Association
5155 Spectrum Way
Unit 3
Mississauga, ON
L4W 5A1
(905) 282-9980
(905) 282-9982 (fax)

RESOURCES FOR THE HOCKEY TRAINER

In the United States, hockey trainers are on their own when it comes to first-aid courses and trainer certificates. USA Hockey does not organize any such educational program. The American Sports Education Program, however, does offer a course on sports first aid.

In Canada, contact the CHA (see above) or your local hockey association. Information on how to contact your provincial association follows. Any of these organizations can inform you on how to go about getting trainer certification.

American Sports Education Program
P.O. Box 5076
Champaign, IL
61825-5076
1-800-747-5698

Hockey Centres of Excellence

In Canada the Hockey Centres of Excellence offer development programs and serve as resource centers for coaching, officiating and sports medicine. (They have no counterpart in the United States.)

British Columbia:
General Motors Place
800 Griffiths Way
Vancouver, BC
V6B 6G1
(604) 899-7770
(604) 899-7771 (fax)

Western:
Box 1060, Olympic Saddledome
Calgary, AB
T2P 2K8
(403) 777-3642
(403) 777-3641 (fax)

Ontario:
Maple Leaf Gardens*
60 Carlton St.
Toronto, ON
M5B 1L1
(416) 408-0039
(416) 408-0053 (fax)
*relocating; new location unconfirmed at press time

Quebec:
Centre Molson
1275 Rue St. Antoine O.
Montreal, QC
H3C 5H8
(514) 925-2240
(514) 652-6641 (fax)

Atlantic:
125 Station St.
St. John, NB
E2L 4X4
(506) 652-2263
(506) 652-6641 (fax)

Halls of Fame

Hockey Hall of Fame
30 Yonge St.
Toronto, ON
M5E 1X8
(416) 360-7765
(416) 360-4622

US Hockey Hall of Fame
801 Hat Trick Ave.
P.O. Box 657
Eveleth, MN
55734
(218) 744-5167
(218) 744-2590 (fax)

Websites

These four sites are a great place to start for general hockey information. They will likely have most anything you need, and they also have extensive lists of hockey-related links.

USA Hockey—www.usahockey.com
The Canadian Hockey Association—www.canadianhockey.com
Hockey Development Centre Ontario—www.hdco.on.ca
Ontario Women's Hockey Association—www.owha.on.ca

And there's also a site that is dedicated to teaching hockey to young players—www.hockeycoach.com

Videos

Fun and Games on Ice
Produced by the Canadian Hockey Association. Packed with great ideas to make learning fun.

The Right Start to Checking
Also by the Canadian Hockey Association, this one covers the skills involved in checking.

The Right Start to Puck Control
The CHA. This video looks at stick-handling, passing, receiving a pass, and shooting.

The Right Start to Skating
The CHA. This introduction to skating covers balance, speed and agility.

Smart Hockey with Mike Bossy
A great video about ways to avoid neck injuries.

All these videos are available from Breakaway, the Official Store of Canadian Hockey, 1-800-441-0449 or (416) 748-5613.

Educational Books

Coaching: The Art and the Science (1997, Dave Chambers, Key Porter Books)
A great book on how to coach hockey. It runs the gamut from drills to sport psychology.

Coaching Youth Hockey (1996, American Sport Education Program, Human Kinetics)
For coaches, especially those coaching kids from 6 to 14.

The Father of Russian Hockey: Tarasov (1997, Anatoly Tarasov, USA Hockey)
Do you think creativity and hockey don't go together? Read this book. It traces the history and evolution of Russian hockey, through the eyes of one of the game's greatest coaches.

The Game (1983, Ken Dryden, Macmillan of Canada)
An inside look at hockey from one of the all-time great goalies.

Hockey: Basics for Beginners (1994, Laurie Work and Scot Ritchie, Kids Can Press)
A small picture book that you can read to your very young child.

The Hockey Coach's Manual: A Guide to Drills, Skills and Conditioning (1997, Michael A. Smith, Firefly Books)
Michael A. Smith is the former General Manager of the Toronto Maple Leafs, and this is one of his several excellent books on coaching hockey.

Hockey Goaltending (1998, Brian Daccord, Human Kinetics)
A complete guide for ice and in-line hockey goalies, for coaches and for parents.

Hockey the NHL Way/Goaltending (1997, Dean Rossiter, Greystone Books)
Tricks of the trade from the greatest modern goalies. Good to read with your child.

Incredible Hockey Drill Book (1994, Dave Chambers, Key Porter Books)
For many coaches this is the bible.

Official Rule Book of the Canadian Hockey Association (yearly, CHA)
If you want to be a coach or a referee in Canada, you can start studying this one now.

Official Rules of Ice Hockey (yearly, USA Hockey)
If you want to be a coach or a referee in the United States, here is your new bible.

The Puck Starts Here (1996, Garth Vaughan, Four East Publications)
A fascinating look at the history and origins of hockey. Fun to read, with great photos.

She Shoots, She Scores (1998, Barbara Stewart, Doubleday Canada)
Women and hockey. A must if you have a girl in the game.

So Your Son Wants to Play in the NHL (1998, Dan and Jay Bylsma, Sleeping Bear Press)
A great book that teaches "hockey parents about life," not just about hockey.

Sport Parent (1994, American Sport Education Program, Human Kinetics)
Should be required reading for all parents with kids in sports.

Strength Training for Young Athletes (1993, Dr. W. Kraemer and Dr. S. Fleck, Human Kinetics)
A sensible approach to the once-controversial subject.

Youth Sports and Self-Esteem (1993, Darrell J. Burnett, Ph.D., Masters Press)
The book to read about building self-esteem. It will change your attitude.

Some Fiction Titles

Here are five great tales, filled with wonderful pictures, to spur your child on to the joys of hockey. The second title is for children to read on their own and is about a girl playing on an all-boys' team.

The Final Game (1997, William Brownridge, ORCA Books)

Hat Trick (1998, Jacqueline Guest, James Lorimer & Co.)

The Hockey Sweater (1979, Roch Carrier, Tundra Books)

The Moccasin Goalie (1995, William Brownridge, ORCA Books)

My Leafs Sweater (1998, Mike Leonetti, Raincoast Books)

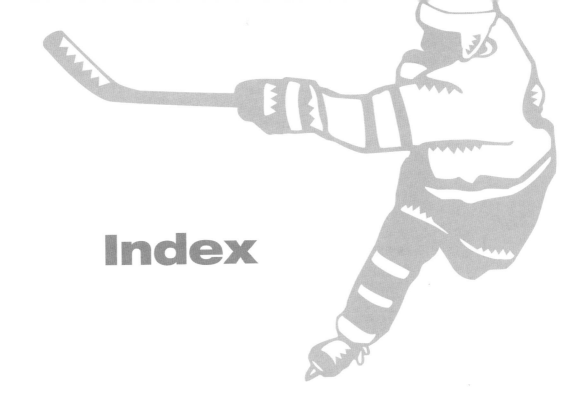

Index

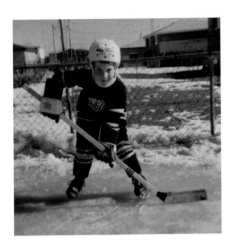

GARY ABRAHAM, M.D.

Gary Abraham played hockey as a child, concluding his hockey career as a winger at university. After taking his medical degree, he specialized in sports medicine and now practices in Brampton, Ontario. He is team physician to junior-A teams and is affiliated with the Toronto Maple Leafs. Dr. Abraham also runs his own hockey school, referees, coaches PeeWee hockey and is a parent of three young hockey players. For him, the game is less about competitiveness and more about fun and self-esteem for young players.